KATE is 49 and has lived in Bahrain since 1995. She works with her husband, Mike, and together they are responsible for the maintenance and care of a large, private psittacine collection of over 800 birds. Kate has had relevant articles printed in editions of *Just Parrots* and *Cage & Aviary Birds*.

Having two grown-up children and a grandchild, her interests include blogging (www.pssitacineanothers.blogspot.com), writing, reading and learning to horse ride and play golf.

MAGGIE is 47, originates from Sweden, and moved to Bahrain in 1983 and married Mohamed.

Although nursing was her chosen career, her interest in animals has led to Maggie becoming involved in different animal societies, and she has had relevant canine articles published in local magazines in Bahrain.

Having no children of her own is not a problem as she shares in the joy of her sister's, brothers', and friends' families.

Her interests are more or less the same as Kate's, but she admits that she is not too good at blogging.

KATE AND MAGGIE have been friends for a number of years, and find that they work well together, as they complement each other's strengths, and any weaknesses can be worked through.

With this in mind, they set up an advice-based web page, www.what-do-we-know.co.uk but did not feel this was enough when it came to certain issues, and this is, in part, how *Quintessential Woman* came to be written.

Quintessential
WOMAN

Quintessential WOMAN

Kate Gammond
&
Maggie Andersson

ATHENA PRESS
LONDON

QUINTESSENTIAL WOMAN
Copyright © Kate Gammond & Maggie Andersson 2007

All Rights Reserved

No part of this book may be reproduced in any form
by photocopying or by any electronic or mechanical means,
including information storage or retrieval systems,
without permission in writing from both the copyright
owner and the publisher of this book.

ISBN 10-digit: 1 84748 116 7
ISBN 13-digit: 978 1 84748 116 0

*Every effort has been made to trace the copyright holders
of works quoted within this book and obtain permission
The publisher apologises for any omissions and is
happy to make necessary changes in subsequent print runs.*

First Published 2007 by
ATHENA PRESS
Queen's House, 2 Holly Road
Twickenham TW1 4EG
United Kingdom

Printed for Athena Press

Contents

Introduction

It is not as if the menopause is a new phenomenon, and the information in this book can be found elsewhere. What we are hoping to have achieved is a different look at the menopause from the 'street level', meaning we are not super women, we don't run companies and we are not selling you a potion that will turn your life around overnight. The menopause came into our lives a bit unexpectedly, and as the majority of our friends are around the same age, the 'change' has been a major topic of conversation and confusion.

Menopause is a changing phenomenon; not so very long ago, women did not live to the age where they would experience infertility. Lifespans were shorter and there was a greater chance of dying before, during or soon after childbirth. Illnesses such as TB, polio and even the flu virus took the lives of so many. As women's life expectancy became longer, the menopause was seen as an illness and treated as such, which more or less brings us up to date. The menopause, we now know, is a natural progression of ageing.

We, the 'baby boomer' generation, are better informed and with improved healthcare can expect to live to the age of eighty-plus.

In this book, we will have a look at the symptoms, from 'what if feels like' to the biological reasons, as well as discussing a woman's well-being and our coming years. As we are more positive and younger in our outlook, the face and concept of old age is changing, and this is what we have addressed in *Quintessential Woman*.

Quintessential Woman

QUINTESSENCE: the pure concentrated essence of anything;
the most essential part, form or embodiment of anything.

Chambers Dictionary, 10th edition[1]

In ancient philosophy, 'quintessence' was thought to be the fifth and highest essence after earth, wind, fire and water, and considered the substance of heavenly bodies.

No, not our words; the above is the meaning as given in our dictionary, and how appropriate – how beautifully the word describes women over 40!

Look at yourself – not in the mirror, but through your mind's eye; look deep enough and without contempt. Who do you see? A woman experienced in life; mature, mischievous, confident, outlandish, extreme, loving, forgiving, exotic, nurturing, eccentric, graceful, proud. As we said: quintessential woman.

Look what you have to offer: a lifetime of adventures; the highs, the lows and all of the in-betweens, and you are all of these things. Celebrate who you are and be thankful that the journey is nowhere near over; there is so much more you can be. Whether in a small way or by taking a huge step, you can face the future because of the past you have experienced.

The one thing that shone through on the questionnaire was that life was for living and there is so much more to do, see and be. Rejoice in being positive and having goals to achieve, mountains to climb... in being a modern-day Boadicea.

---

[1] Chambers Harrap Publishers Ltd, 2006.

Change-a-Pause

Believe in You

Always follow your heart
You can fly and you can soar
You can open any door
You can sail the widest ocean
You can set the wheels in motion
'Cause dreamers come through
If you just start
By simply listening to your heart
Just dream and do believe in you.

Author unknown

Have you ever had one of those mornings when you have dark circles around the eyes and your skin is dull, the wrinkles seem more prominent and the greying temples remind you of how old you are? Well, you can feel sorry for yourself and have a miserable day, or look yourself in the eye and tell yourself what a wonderful woman you are!

Menstruation, pregnancy and menopause unite women the world over regardless of colour, creed, religion or status, and, whether you live in a third-world country or the cosmopolitan Western societies, these life changes occur at around the same ages for all of us. Some of us will have been lucky enough to live a life with choices, and many, many others will have had a hard life that will have aged them prematurely. Sisterhood should have no boundaries and hormones are universal!

We liked this comment by Gerard M DiLeo: 'Just a few generations ago, most women fell into one of three categories:

pregnant, breastfeeding or dead', meaning that women did not experience menopause because they did not live long enough, and even a hundred years ago, according to Dr Annie Evans, a specialist in women's health at the Bristol Royal Infirmary, 'the average age of the menopause was 47, but the life expectancy of British women was only 49.' We are the lucky ones; due to better living conditions, ample food and health care, we are living longer. Our generation of women can now expect to spend up to a third of their lives post-menopause.

What is menopause? Menopause comes from the Greek words '*meno pausis*'; *meno* is 'month' and *pausis* is 'end'. You may also know it as 'the change of life'. It signifies the time in a woman's life when the ovaries no longer release a monthly egg cell; menstruation ceases, and your natural childbearing years are over.

So, if you have not had a period for one year (for women over 50) or two years (for women under 50), you are post-menopausal. If you are still menstruating and suffering from any of the symptoms associated with the onset of menopause, you are said to be peri-menopausal, and this is the body's way of preparing you for the menopause.

Confusing, isn't it?

The time it takes from the first symptoms to being post-menopause can vary from two to fifteen years. The onset of peri-menopause symptoms starts between the ages of 35 and 45, and in some cases even earlier. This is a natural process and, we think, one of the most significant phases in a woman's life. Knowledge empowers you to make informed choices, and these choices, hopefully, enable you to manage any symptoms that you may be experiencing.

What if you are not in the above age group? Premature menopause has many causes, such as surgical menopause, medical menopause and premature ovarian failure (POF). All are drastic for women who are diagnosed in their early twenties, as they will have little chance of conceiving naturally, if at all.

Surgical menopause may be caused by a hysterectomy, which involves the complete removal of the uterus except for the cervix; with this operation, you retain the ovaries. Your menstruation will stop, and menopause symptoms may come at the same age as they would normally, or, in rare cases, at a younger age.

With bilateral oophorectomy, both of the ovaries are removed, and in some cases both procedures are performed at the same time (total abdominal hysterectomy with bilateral salpingo-oophorectomy – isn't that a mouthful?). This means that you will lose most of your body's natural production of oestrogen and progesterone, which is not to be taken lightly. If you have had both procedures, you will cease to menstruate and you will start to experience the peri-menopausal symptoms more or less immediately.

Medical menopause can occur when you are administered treatment such as chemotherapy; you may go into either temporary or permanent menopause. Anti-cancer medication can also damage the ovaries, reducing the amounts of hormones they produce, which can lead to irregular menstruation cycles or infertility. Before making any decision on the above, ask questions; make sure you know the facts and the likely outcome of your treatment. Contact support groups. Remember, this is your body, your choice and your right.

Signs and symptoms of peri-menopause:

- trouble sleeping
- hot flushes, night sweats, cold flushes, clammy feeling
- joint ache
- loss of interest in sex
- irregular heartbeat
- mood swings, sudden tears
- irregular menstruation
- dry vagina

- crashing fatigue
- anxiety
- difficulty in concentrating; disorientation; mental confusion
- memory lapses
- incontinence, e.g. while laughing, sneezing
- crawly, itchy skin
- increased tension in muscles
- breast tenderness
- headaches
- indigestion, flatulence, gas pain, nausea
- bloated feeling
- allergy increase
- weight gain
- hair loss on body, but increase in facial hair
- light-headedness, dizziness, loss of balance
- body odour changes
- tingling in the arms and legs
- bleeding in the gums, bad taste in mouth, bad breath, mouth ulcers
- fingernails softer and crack or break easily
- ringing in the ears (tinnitus), whooshing, buzzing, etc.
- osteoporosis
- depression

No wonder depression figures on the list – by the time you have finished evaluating all of the other symptoms, of course that's how you feel! Blame it on the hormones (or should it be 'her moans'?). First, we had to go through puberty when our hormones, namely testosterone, oestrogen, progesterone and follicle-stimulating hormone (FSH), produced in the pituitary gland, kicked in. Do you remember when you stood in front of the mirror, looking at those two small and painful bumps on your chest? Sadly, for some of us, those pert little breasts are now two semi-deflated bags!

These two stages represent our 'rite of passage' into womanhood as well as our fertile decline, and in both we experience physical, mental and emotional changes. But now our sex hormones, oestrogen and progesterone, two of the hormones controlling your monthly cycle, are doing an about-turn, and the pituitary gland responds by producing more FSH. Please remember, any of the symptoms above can have a number of medical reasons, and doctors may check your hormone levels to determine whether the symptoms you are experiencing can be attributed to the 'change'. There are also tests now available that can give you reliable information regarding your fertility; these tests are aimed as a guide for women who are looking to conceive as well as giving an indication regarding the onset of menopause.

The natural life of the ovaries is approximately thirty-five years. Let us say that you started to menstruate at the age of twelve; that means that you should be in menopause at the age of 48. That was easy, yes? But not so reliable, as the eggs in our ovaries are like small grains of sand: at birth, we have several hundred thousand; when we reach puberty and menstruation starts, we are down to about 300,000, and by the age of 37 we have 25,000 eggs left, give or take. At the menopause stage, we are left with around 1,000 eggs; as you can see, the number of eggs rapidly decreases.

Can the doctor really count the eggs? No, he can't, but he can measure the ovarian volume. So, if they measure the ovarian volume (ovaries shrinks as we age) and do a transvaginal ultrasound, they should be able to predict the time when menopause will set in and for how many more years you will be fertile.

Another test available, via a blood sample, is the anti-Müllerian hormone test. This hormone (AMH) is in part responsible for the production of oestrogen, and the test, which measures the ovarian function, is considered to be an accurate indicator of a woman's fertility as well as a method of determining the approach and onset of menopause. This test can also be used to judge the possible success of IVF treatment and to measure the extent of polycystic ovarian failure (PCOS).

With these tests, women who are opting to become first-time mothers later in life will have the chance to keep a check on their fertility and plan accordingly. Hopefully, women of tomorrow will have more information available and, due to advances in medicine, learn more about how their body and 'body clock' is working.

Some women will go through the menopause with hardly any problems at all; menstruation literally stops overnight with few, if any, symptoms. Just who are these women? Are their hormones different or are they more resilient? Do we applaud them or hate them? Well, that depends on the kind of day we are having.

Let's be honest: we women do not even think about the onset of menopause until we are experiencing the symptoms, and why should we? Most of us are still in denial about being in the 40-plus age group – middle-aged! Even if we have thought about these changes, have heard the horror stories and are feeling rather smug (surely, when our time comes to go through the 'change', we will sail through; well, it's not an illness, is it?), the smiles are soon wiped off our faces. The reality, for some, is very different, and, if possible, it is always a good idea to ask your mum or older sisters how it was for them; it may give you an insight into what's in store for you!

Do factors such as culture, environment, nutrition, etc., play a part? More of that later…

Mental Fog

★ SMILE TIME ★

Lord, help me to remember that nothing is going to happen to
me today that you and I together cannot handle.

Dear Lord,
So far today I've done all right.
I have not gossiped.
I have not lost my temper, lied or cheated.
I haven't been greedy, grumpy, nasty, selfish or overindulgent.
I am very thankful for that.
But in a few minutes, Lord, I am going to get out of bed, and
from that moment on I am going to need a lot more help.

Anonymous

If you can't quite remember when things started to change, don't worry; you are experiencing a stage that many women go through. You may become forgetful and feel confused or overwhelmed by situations that, once upon a time, you could take in your stride. Keeping track of a conversation involving more than two people seems a task in itself, and the name of a close friend, at times, eludes you. Your mood swings may become erratic and you are tearful for no apparent reason; it feels like a permanent state of PMS, and, coupled with poor concentration, you feel as though you are losing your self-control and sanity. The world has turned upside down and you don't know why.

It is a relief to find out that the symptoms that you are experiencing are due to the onset of the menopause rather than early-onset Alzheimer's! This is your body's way of preparing you for the menopause, and, now that you know the cause, you can start to comprehend what is happening. You have to come to terms with this phase in your life, like it or not.

Emotionally, we are on a roller coaster and we often assume that depression enters our lives because of 'external' worries; maybe we are not happy with our partner, job and home life, or life in general. This, of course, is true, and we are sure that all of us at some point will suffer or have suffered from a bout of depression. It is no secret that women tend to suffer more than men, but we are talking about a depression that can be attributed to the chemical changes going on within our bodies, which affect the neurotransmitters in the brain. How many times have you heard women say they don't know why they are depressed, as, in theory, everything is great and they couldn't ask for more?

Well, if you have ongoing depression or a feeling of sadness that now seems to be a permanent part of your life, it is treatable, and, with all the physical and emotional changes happening in and to your body, this is one extra weight that you do not need to carry around. It is enough dealing with any of the symptoms associated with the 'change' without their being compounded by depression. Do not be ashamed or feel a failure because you seek professional help; depression can cast a cloud in many areas of your life and, left untreated, only deepens. The more you have to cope with, the harder it becomes. Consider what a day is like for so many women: they go to work and care for a family and the home, and, let's face it, both kids and hubbies tend to rely on them to make sure their clothes are washed and meals are cooked, the homework is done and on and on… 'molehills' that you could have taken in your stride once now become 'mountains'.

You really do need to put yourself first, because if you don't, you will feel as though your world is crumbling around you. How can you take care of the other things in your life if you haven't taken care of yourself? Pay a visit to your doctor and receive the help you need; depression is an illness, and, with the right treatment, you will feel as though that weight has been lifted from you. Be selfish, not selfless; there are no medals awarded for this job!

Something for you to consider are women who see the menopause as an illness and use the symptoms to control family and friends. They will always have an excuse for not doing something or for being snappy and argumentative, and, though they may dabble in different remedies, none are ever right for them. Sadly, these women may have always been self-absorbed – the world revolves around them or it doesn't revolve at all! The one thing they should not do is let life pass them by because of ego. There are probably more underlying problems than they are willing to admit to, and, if they can seek help, life will be richer than they ever dared to imagine, and family and friends will be supportive when they can see a positive personality emerging, especially if that person has let their guard down on occasions to reveal the real woman they are. Yes menopause can make you feel ill, but spending two to ten years or more milking the symptoms only makes you the loser. The hardest step to take is the very first one, but if you can take it, either on your own or with help, you will only go forward.

Body Talk

You may think we have a strange sense of humour and that we are making fun of you – we are not. A lot of what follows has been experienced either by us or by our close friends; we have listened to each other, commiserated with each other, supported when support was needed, shed tears… Do you know what gets you through troubled times more than anything else? Laughter – being able to laugh at yourself – and, of course, friendship.

There is a vague line you have crossed without even realising it until you look in the mirror; who the hell is that looking back at you? Rod Stewart's 'Maggie May' comes to mind: 'the morning sun when it's in your face really shows your age'. Denial is the first option, along with covering up every mirror. Well, you don't need the mirror to tell you things are changing

– everything is heading south: the eyelids, jowls, breast and bum, even the arches on your feet! And just what are those 'bat-wings' under your arms?

It is not as though it happened overnight, and we are sure that not everyone suffers the same consequences. It's the little things that catch your attention: the once engaging laughter lines around the eyes, remember? Your significant other said how they made your eyes sparkle; they are now a permanent feature and have gone from engaging to permanently engraved! It probably has something to do with squinting while trying to read your horoscope at arm's length in the daily paper – which, of course, means stronger lenses in your glasses. And just where did you put them?

The sprinkling of grey that was once enhanced by high-lights or a semi-permanent tint is now in need of a full-on monthly retouch of those telltale roots! Eyebrows are tweaked a little more to get rid of the white flecks, and – shock horror! – the pubes are greying... Well, a 'Mexican' sorts that out; make sure the razor is sharp and that you don't apply the wax in the wrong places.

On a good day, we have the vitality to change the world, and on a bad day, the unknown aches and pains that plague our body are a sure sign of a major, life-threatening illness. The knees and knuckles begin to stiffen and creak and, hell's bells, you even start to walk with care in case you fall. Watch those hips, girls – Zimmer frames are just around the corner...

The words 'flight or fight' take on a new meaning: half way through the weekly shop – you are wondering how you will make it to the cash till, wait in line and then go through the motions of unloading your trolley, paying for your goods and reloading them when all you want to do is run away to some safe place where you do not have to fight for your breath. Welcome to the mysterious and unpredictable world of panic attacks, thanks to your adrenaline system.

Late nights and early mornings no longer mix, and, if you

have managed a late night, regardless of the fact that you haven't had a drink, why do you have a hangover the following day?

You even start to sound like your mother. 'Would you like to go out for a meal?' 'Well, OK, as long as we don't eat too late; I can't go to bed on a full stomach – acid indigestion…'

It no longer surprises us that we can sustain an in-depth conversation on bloatedness and constipation and the possible remedies when out with the girls for a coffee – and that is a low-fat decaf cappuccino, by the way; can't be doing with the palpitations and anxiety due to a caffeine rush.

And, for goodness' sake, don't get into any 'cat fights'; with all the cracking, flaking and chipping of your nails, you would certainly lose.

Things do get worse: coughing, sneezing and laughing can be a major embarrassment when the bladder is full, and let's not forget the night sweats, hot flushes and the 'crawling skin' sensation. You are either getting out of bed soaked, in need of a shower and a change of bedding, or you are jumping out of bed, convinced you are being attacked by an army of ants!

And so to bed… oh, we forgot to mention the 'unmentionables': a lack of natural lubricant in the vagina, the slackening vaginal muscles and sex drive. Some days you will be an insatiable raging nympho and at other times you will ask, 'What sex drive?'

And while we are on the subject, don't forget to check the tube of KY, the one in the drawer by the bed; has it gone past its sell-by date? Put it on your shopping list; you will find it between hair products and aftershave. Spontaneity is a thing of the past.

Then there is the sleeping problem, or should we say a problem in sleeping? No matter how tired you are when you climb into bed, thirty minutes later you are wide awake. You spend half the night tossing and turning and watching the hands on the clock tick away well into early morning. Counting sheep and deep relaxation no longer work, and by 4 a.m. you regret that you did not get up hours earlier, make yourself that cup of tea and read a chapter or two of your book, catch up on some correspondence or watch some late-night soaps on TV.

Even if you did manage a good night's sleep and you get up feeling all is well with the world, you didn't count on someone taking out your batteries, did you? That is how it feels: you are busy getting on with your day, when *whoosh*, your 'get-up-and-go' has got up and gone and you need to either sit down or, if at home, crawl back to bed until the feeling passes.

Then you get to thinking, if you are like this at 40-something, what will you be like at 70? Your mind wanders off to some point in the future, panic ensues and the vertigo and tinnitus are only confirmation that life is spiralling out of control… along with your sense of balance.

Can it get worse? A word of *caution*: something we hear about is 'menopause babies'. What are the chances of becoming pregnant during peri-menopause? Sorry, girls, it is possible if you are still ovulating – even if it is irregular. It only takes one determined spermatozoa and no contraception, and that puts paid to a quiet retirement and the accompanying nest egg.

In spite of these challenges, midlife is often a satisfying time. Ah! The pleasures of being mature. Is there hope? Can you be saved? Read on…

Sexual Dysfunction

Below is an article by Dr Gerard M DiLeo, MD, FACOG, which we think is relevant when it comes to assessing one of the possible underlying causes of sexual dysfunction.

As women get older, menopause becomes inevitable. Oestrogen, widely considered *the* female hormone, falls and is eventually absent. Progesterone, the *other* female hormone, likewise falls victim to menopause. What most people don't realise is that yet another female hormone, testosterone, will fall as well.

Both men and women have testosterone. But since men have so much more of it, it is mistakenly called the male hormone. We know what testosterone does for a woman by what happens when it's gone: sex drive, or libido, suffers. Here are some interesting observations about menopause, testosterone, libido and quality of life:

- Testosterone either declines by 50% or is absent altogether in women after the menopause. The adrenal glands can provide some, but this source is very unreliable after menopause.

- With a fall in testosterone, libido falls and, with it, frequency of sexual intimacy.

- With a fall in sexual frequency, more arguments occur in a marriage and partners grow more distant, increasing estrangement, either through separation psychologically or separation of actual addresses.

- With lifespans lasting longer than ever, and with the baby boomers in the menopausal years, we can expect an 'epidemic' of loss of sexual function and happiness.

Is this putting too much importance on sex? The answer is 'no' in the strongest possible terms. You don't have to be Masters and Johnson to know that sex pervades our lives. All of the media is absolutely obsessed with it. But this is a charade: actually, all of the media are obsessed with money, and since sex sells… there you are. But sex sells because we are the ones obsessed. Is this nasty or vile or debauched? No, again.

We are deeply sexual beings, and to deny it is as ridiculous as denying hunger or thirst or the need for camaraderie, friendship or love. And the statistics on sexual dysfunction and marital discord after the menopause prove this. Sexual dysfunction is a real pathology that needs to be treated. In menopausal women, the first need that should be addressed is the oestrogen. Oestrogen provides structural nourishment for the vaginal tissue, lubricating glands and the clitoris. Decreased sensitivity of the clitoris occurs with decreased oestrogen. More importantly, with its absence, the thinning vaginal walls may lead to painful intercourse, which then adds a severe psychological obstacle to overcome in regaining a normal intimacy between the married couple.

A trial of oestrogen replacement, besides addressing a possible cause of sexual dysfunction, will also provide the benefits of reducing the risk of heart disease and osteoporosis. (Progesterone should be added, too, in the presence of the uterus, so that a balanced effect on this tissue will prevent any precancerous changes in the uterus.) Once oestrogen deficits have been corrected, if there is inadequate improvement in libido, testosterone should be added, which is the whole point of this article.

One of the problems that women have is the prejudice against their gender when it comes to vague complaints like decreased libido. Male and female doctors alike have been traditionally prone to ignore these complaints as being 'all in the head'. This attitude has been unfairly strengthened by the fact that women outnumber men in depression by 2:1 and in anxiety by 4:1. But I've always found that it's the ethically correct thing to give a woman the benefit of the doubt before writing off a complaint as irrationally neurotic. To do so is a tragic misdiagnosis that is disgraceful to the medical pro-fession. But along with the care of not labelling complaints as hysterical, a physician must also be aware that there may in fact be some psychological factors that are part (not the only cause) of the problem. In this vein, a psychologist or social worker can be helpful in rounding out the treatment.

But if the only problem is hormonal, then this can be diagnosed… and corrected. Quality of life depends on it, and so too may the marriage.[2]

---

[2] www.gynob.com.

The above is very true, though, statistically, it is said that women over 40 are in their prime when it comes to sex. Is that true? Well, if you are one of those women then way to go, girl! How do others see themselves? How many times have we heard women, not necessarily older, saying things like, 'Oh, I'm past all "that" now', or 'We don't do "that" any more'; or even 'Later in life, you will find a good book more satisfying than sex', and 'Oh, we have separate beds/bedrooms'. The list goes on. Did these women ever enjoy sex? Are they ignorant of satisfying their or their partner's sexual needs? Do they no longer find their partner physically attractive, or did they fall out of love? Is there a medical reason? There are so many questions.

The one thing that can be said is that there is no such thing as a 'normal' sex drive; having less or more sexual desire than your partner does not mean that you are having a problem, only that there is a difference in how you both relate to your sexual needs and frequency.

Let's face it: for some couples, to communicate their needs and sexual preferences with each other is totally taboo, and a lot of couples never regain the intimacy they once had, nor do they want to. Maybe your partner is also relieved that he no longer has to perform – it cuts both ways.

This can also be the point in your lives when your relationship comes under strain, and this can lead to you or your partner seeking solace, change or excitement elsewhere. Is this understandable? Possibly. Is it forgivable? This will depend on the strength of your relationship, and how you both see the future and with whom.

What if you have always had a full and healthy sex life and you are now no longer interested? Do you feel resentful or relieved? Or has this problem gone on for so long that you do not know how to overcome it? Do you feel less attractive and think this is how your partner sees you? What do you do when a previously healthy sexual relationship all but disappears?

It helps if you have someone to talk to, especially if that 'someone' is your partner. If your sexual appetite has diminished, you both need to know why and you will both need reassurance. There is nothing to stop you sitting down together, having a heart-to-heart over a glass of wine or a cup of tea or simply holding hands. Gaining a connection is what matters, and these acts, although seemingly small, are ones of intimacy. Look back, take time to reflect and see if there has been a pattern to your sexual decline. If there is no stress between you, of the 'your fault – no, your fault' kind, look at how you have been feeling and why. Do you feel tired or depressed, unattractive because of weight gain or because you 'feel' older? Maybe you still feel sexy inside, but from the outside you can only see yourself as ageing. You may not want to be intimate because you don't become aroused as easily, and the night sweats and the hot flushes really are a turn-off; the only fire you are experiencing is one that leaves you drenched in your own sweat and not wanting to be touched, and women, so often, feel like failures in the bedroom.

If you still find your partner attractive and want to get things back on track, it may be a case of your hormones playing havoc with your life. Your sex drive can be lower; the vagina may be dry and less flexible because of the natural thinning of the lining, and, due to the lack of natural lubrication, intercourse can be painful. Sometimes, it is the little things that can be easily put right; if intercourse is uncomfortable, it may be just a case of using a lubricant or a vaginal hormone cream.

Otherwise, female sexual dysfunction is recognised and can be treated. There are a number of reasons for a woman to lose interest in sex, such as:

- stress

- relationship problems and boredom

- surgery

- low self-esteem
- menopause
- hormonal imbalance
- exhaustion
- depression.

Speak to your doctor, a marriage guidance counsellor or a therapist; sometimes all you need is to talk and be heard! There are solutions to these problems.

Once you have found and understood the reason you feel the way you do, with help and support and the will to make your relationship work, when you are ready to be intimate, lovemaking will again be physically and emotionally rewarding for you and your partner. It has long been understood that sexual intercourse and love have very little to do with each other, but 'lovemaking' is the icing on the cake. If your relationship is strong, it will withstand this hiccup. Until that time, share other intimacies and look forward to the future.

Nowadays, we appear to be under the numbers' spell; sexual performance for women as well as men is counted in the terms of 'how many times' per day, week or month, and, with the emergence of the 'little blue pill', quality has bowed to quantity. The sad fact is that Viagra does not always solve the impotency problem and, interestingly, there are many couples who choose to be celibate within a marriage, though they do still maintain a close and loving relationship; love and intimacy have many facets, and age should not impose limitations on love or how you choose to express your love.

Internal Furnace

'Is it me or is it hot in here?' How many times have you said these words or heard them uttered? They have many names: hot flushes, power surges or night sweats. Did you know that about 85% of women suffer from mild to severe bouts during the peri-menopause and menopause stage? They seemingly come from nowhere; you have no control over them, and they can happen at any time. One minute, you feel quite normal, then, suddenly, you start to feel the sometimes intense heat along with the sweat that starts to break out on the forehead, scalp, between your breasts and even as far down as your hands. Panic ensues, and how embarrassed you feel during those meetings, dinners out, etc., when they start; of course, they always seem to surface when you are out in public. Where is that fan? You become anxious, possibly experiencing palpitations or even panic attack and you are sure that everyone is staring at you. Your body odour, at these times, can smell distinctly 'fishy', possibly due to the hormones changing, and the more you panic on the inside the worse it gets.

It is easy to say 'don't do anything drastic', because all you want to do is take flight, but if you just wait it out, keeping yourself as calm as possible while keeping your breathing slow and regular, it will only take a few seconds to several minutes before it is over, even though, we know, it feels like hours. It can help if you dress in layers so you can remove clothing to help you feel cooler.

Researchers are not really sure how these hot flushes come about; there are many different theories. One is that the temperature system, controlled by the hypothalamus gland, can be the trigger, and it is also possible there may be a direct link between the loss of oestrogen and hypothalamus gland.

Hot flushes are a common symptom at the peri-menopause stage, but the good news (is it?) is that they are normal.

Metabolism

It is a fact that, as women age, they tend to gain weight, and we hear things like 'I have a slow metabolism' or 'it's the hormones'. This, in a roundabout way, is true – but it is not an excuse.

'Metabolism' actually refers to the numerous chemical processes going on in your body, and the BMR, basal metabolic rate, is the amount of energy your body needs to maintain itself. The metabolic rate can be influenced by gender, muscle-to-fat ratio and age, though metabolism does vary from person to person, and guess what: the metabolic rate of a man tends to be higher than that of a woman, because they are usually larger and have less body fat – up to 10% less! Make sure he knows this the next time he moans about your love handles!

Other reasons for a slowing metabolism include faulty genes; these can affect the metabolism by causing problems such as fructose intolerance, galactosaemia and phenylketonuria (PKU).

A diet that is high in saturated fats and sugars is of no help at all, and then, of course, we come to the good old hormones. Hypothyroidism (an underactive thyroid) and hyperthyroidism (an overactive thyroid) are just two of many hormonal disorders, and, luckily, thyroid dysfunction, once diagnosed, can be treated.

Anxiety can also contribute to how our metabolism performs. We are sure you have heard people say 'she lives on her nerves' – well, living on her nerves burns up the calories!

We also lose muscle as we get older, because we are not usually as physically active, and the phrase 'use it or lose it' applies, because muscle turns to fat. Most women experience a change in their weight and shape as they age; apparently, it's OK to be pear-shaped, but not an apple shape. We are talking about the toxic fat around the middle, that ever-increasing 'spare tyre' and a waist measurement over 31.5 inches, for women, is a warning sign. Apparently, for every two pounds gained during menopause, the risk of high blood pressure increases by 5%, and carrying this kind of fat around can also lead to strokes, heart disease and diabetes, to name but a few. Depressing, isn't it? We are being hit left, right and centre – sex is off and the weight is on!

Even if we try to lose weight, many of us become dis-heartened. We are eating less, and either our weight remains the same or there is just a small loss when we step onto the scales. The reason for this is that our body thinks we are experiencing a famine, so the BMR slows in order to save your energy.

You can't control your metabolism, but you can make it work for you by exercising, and that is why it is important to keep as physically fit as possible; we are talking about the kind of exercise that leaves you a little breathless, at least three thirty-minute sessions a week. If you think about it, before we became temporarily celibate, we could work up that kind of a sweat without even getting out of bed!

If you are not used to exercising or have health problems, *please* see your doctor for advice on exercise and diet regimes. Don't go out there and go mad – we can't afford any court cases!

Help!

When it comes to dealing with any of the symptoms, only you can know how you are feeling. Unless you are really clued up about women's health matters, you will probably be experienc-ing a few of the peri-menopause symptoms on a regular basis before you even realise there could be a problem or a good reason for feeling the way you do. It may cross your mind that how you are feeling could be the onset of the menopause, but usually as a first option, especially if you are in your early to mid-40s, is to dismiss it because you are 'not that age yet'.

'That age', regardless of the number of candles on your birthday cake, now takes you to a new level in your life, and the first thing most of us do is find information about the menopause; most of us haven't learned yet that there is a pre/peri and a post-menopause, but there is plenty of infor-mation available and, surprisingly, it now seems to appear daily in your favourite magazine, newspaper and even the news.

How could you have missed it previously when it is so important? As we said before, you had no reason to look.

So you are now armed with various magazines and books and are ready to embrace or fight this inconvenience in your life. Some women decide there and then that HRT is the path they are going to take, though nowadays you have to convince the doctor that this is what you want, as prescriptions for HRT aren't as readily available as they once were. A doctor should assess your medical history and even that of your close family to make sure there are no reasons for you not to take HRT, and before the prescription is handed over there should be a thorough exam, including a Pap smear, breast check, blood pressure and cholesterol level check as well as checking your weight. Hormone levels should also be checked before you are given HRT so that you can be prescribed the correct dosage of the relevant hormones; this would address any imbalances and avoid overdosing on the hormones that are naturally occurring within the body, which, if you think about it, makes sense. Talk to your doctor about the addition of testosterone if you are suffering from low or no libido; our sex drive should not stop just because we are no longer fertile! Many women are happy with HRT; it suits them, and they have not experienced any problems that have, of late, been associated with taking HRT. Usually, it is the women who suffer from extreme symptoms who benefit the most.

There are plenty of roads to travel when you are looking for alternative ways to manage your symptoms. For a lot of women, it is a wake-up call: your body is telling you things and you should listen. Examine your feelings and how you are, or are not, coping, and try to find a way of dealing with the peri-menopause that allows you to be comfortable within yourself. It may be a case of altering your diet; we all know that certain foods and drinks can cause palpitations, acid indigestion, bloatedness, etc. Others will choose to take supplements specifically designed for women who are premenopause, or other products that have been recommended.

It may be that you need to take a daily time-out – finding a place in your home that is out of bounds for thirty minutes or an hour while you allow yourself to unwind and calm any jagged nerves. Maybe you now find you enjoy taking the dog for a walk; you are out in the fresh air, and you will have a captive audience who will listen to your moans about your day and how you are feeling without giving an opinion or starting an argument. It's surprising how much better we feel when we can get those annoyances off our chest.

Please don't close your family off, especially if you do have children at home; regardless of their ages, explain what is happening and how you are feeling and apologise in advance for the days when you are snappy. They will still, no doubt, get lippy with you, but they will understand. It's a lot better to be able to shout, 'Keep out of my way today; I'm feeling like an unexploded bomb!' than to have your family walking on eggshells because they don't know how you will react to anything.

If you feel that you have pent-up anger, the climbing-the-wall kind, then you need to find a more energetic release that will make you feel at ease with yourself. Consider a dance class: a sexy salsa or an adults' tap class will get rid of that anger, and music is always good for the soul. Or, if at home, turn up the radio and bop around to your heart's content.

Down in the dumps? Watch a favourite movie – it doesn't matter if it makes you laugh or cry as both are good releases – or treat yourself to a massage: let someone else smooth your cares away. Take up tai chi, meditation or yoga; you will find that all your thoughts are put to one side as you concentrate on your breathing or getting your body into the right position.

Any therapy, hobby or sport that takes you 'out of yourself' can make you feel as though you are giving body and soul a break. You will find that the more you concentrate on getting it right, the less you are thinking of 'you'; as any worries or tensions are banished, you start to feel at ease within your body. Do not worry that you feel this way for only a couple of hours a week; as you become more relaxed and confident in what you are doing, you will 'tune in' more easily. It does take effort on your part, but do not force yourself to concentrate or relax or you will be defeating the object, which is to naturally relax. You may also need to try out different classes, therapies and so on to find which suit you. Luckily, most classes will let you join in for a couple of sessions as a 'taster', and then you can choose which new hobby or therapy feels right for you.

Tai chi claims to have many benefits. It:

- oxygenates every cell and muscle in your body
- helps regulate the immune system
- self-massages the internal organs
- increases strength and flexibility
- improves concentration
- increases awareness
- develops better balance and coordination
- strengthens the muscles
- reduces muscular stiffness
- helps to relieve back pain
- produces better relaxation and calm
- improves posture both when still and moving
- assists the digestive system and abdominal organs
- improves circulation
- produces vitality
- is good for arthritis, asthma, diabetes, blood pressure, headache and heart disease.

(Wow!) We can definitely say tai chi improves coordination. When we first started to learn tai chi we literally could not coordinate different parts of our body independently; as a matter of fact, we looked a bit like marionettes who had had their wires cut. With practice, you develop the ability of the left and right sides of your brain to work in harmony and your limbs start looking as if they do belong to you.

Yoga, as most of us know, has been practised for hundreds of years; there are many different forms taught and, as with tai chi, the health benefits are numerous. We think most of us know that yoga can be calming, especially when the different breathing techniques are practised regularly. Learning to calm yourself down and 'keep it together' can be very important, not only to you but those around you, be they family or work colleagues. Long-term stress is harmful and damaging to body and mind, and there are many illnesses that are directly attributed to stress.

If you enjoy having a massage, there are many different types available. Ayurvedic massage, LaStone therapy or an invigorating body scrub can help your body to detoxify, as well as aiding the lymphatic system. Acupressure can help reduce tension and headaches, ease anxiety and help with fatigue; you will feel so pampered and relaxed, and don't you deserve it?

Reiki is another ancient healing method that is widely used, either on its own or in conjunction with crystals. Even in this day and age, a lot of alternative therapies are brushed off as being a bit 'wacko', but we have found that, even if you are initially sceptical, what you can experience, in terms of relaxation of body and mind, will leave you wanting more. If you feel easier within yourself, haven't you achieved what you set out to do – relieve symptoms of the peri-menopause?

As we have previously advised, see a qualified practitioner; ask about their credentials, experience and how long they have been practising. A good practitioner will take the time to ask about your health and lifestyle, and they should keep and respect your confidentiality. They will also advise you to seek medical help if you are having any ongoing health problems, and most doctors do realise the benefits of complementary therapies when it comes to treating the body as a 'whole'.

Even trying an alternative therapy, such as reiki, crystal healing or reflexology can be wonderfully beneficial and totally relaxing. Whatever it is that makes you feel good in yourself and about yourself is always a boost for self-esteem.

One 'remedy' you should avoid is alcohol. It is so easy to pour a glass of wine and, yes, it does take the edge off, but it will take many more glasses in the future to achieve that 'fuzzy' softer edge. Alcoholics are usually the last ones to realise they have a problem, so, if you are tempted to seek solace in a bottle, take our advice and seek help. No one will judge you or consider you to be weak; it takes a strong person to battle the bottle demons. Some facts that you may not know about booze: the recommended fourteen units a week for women is based on a 125 ml glass of 8% volume wine, but most wines are between 12–13% volume and the average glass size is 175 ml. A light drinker, according to the UK Medical Council, is less than six units a week. There are also concerns regarding 'midlife' binge drinkers (do you drink or share a bottle of wine every day?) with respect to the health problems they will incur and the fact that, as we age, our body does not tolerate alcohol in the same way it did when we were younger; that's why you may feel tipsy after only one glass!

There are many, many products available, and, as the pharmaceutical industry progresses and learns more about how our bodies work, it is feasible that, in the future, products may be tailor-made to suit the individual. In the meantime, whether you opt for HRT or a more natural approach to help manage symptoms associated with the menopause, we strongly advise you to do your homework and get the facts on any of the numerous products that are available.

Conventional and alternative products do not always mix,

and alternative products are not necessarily safer than conventional medicine: these can also cause side effects; even vitamins taken in excess can cause a reaction. If you are taking prescription medicine, you must consult with your doctor, pharmacist or alternative practitioner before taking any additional supplements. If you feel your concerns are brushed aside, seek a second opinion, and remember: this is *your* health, *your* decision.

Please remember, with all products, conventional or alternative, what suits one person may not suit you. When reading a label, think: do you know what a 'natural' product is? Did you know that something synthetic can also be natural, while something considered natural may be foreign to the human body? This can be very confusing, and the key here is not whether a compound is natural to plants or animals but is the compound natural to the human body and identical to compounds made by the human body? As an example: medication being used because it is 'natural' for humans is insulin. The 'natural' insulin was taken from cows and pigs to treat diabetics; this animal insulin was 'natural' because it came from a natural source, but the molecular structure was foreign to the human body, and many times human diabetics develop allergic reactions to the 'natural' insulin. Thanks to scientists, diabetics now have a 'human', synthetically-made insulin molecule that is native to the natural human body. So, the next time you read or see the word 'natural' advertised, read the small print.

We take both prescribed medication and alternative remedies, as well as vitamin and mineral supplements; our needs and what we take are different to each other's, and yours will be too, and that is why we will not be recommending a particular product. Below are some of the remedies that women have found beneficial through the different stages of the menopause:

- *HRT* (hormone replacement therapy). Oestrogen and progesterone are the two main supplements used in HRT, and it is available in the form of tablets, skin patches, implants, vaginal pessaries, gels or creams. Controversy surrounds HRT and it has had both positive and negative effects on women.

- *Black cohosh* is contraindicated if you are on HRT, and, if taken long term, you should have a one-month break every six months.

- *Evening primrose oil*. Contraindicated if you are taking blood-thinning medication such as warfarin or aspirin or have temporal lobe epilepsy.

- *Siberian ginseng*. Contraindicated if you are on HRT or taking medication for the heart, or if you have any of the following: schizophrenia, epilepsy, diabetes, high blood pressure. A break of one month is recommended every three months.

- *Soya products*, which contain a type of plant oestrogen. There is a question mark over soya with regard to breast problems.

- *St John's Wort*. Contraindicated if you are taking anti-depressants or drugs such as tetracycline, or have hypersensitivity to sunlight.

- *Valerian*. Contraindicated if you are taking sedatives or drugs which affect the central nervous system.

- *Chaste berry*. Not recommended during pregnancy (well, you never know…)

- *Maca*. High potassium content, therefore not recommended for people with renal problems.

Does this mean that everyone who takes any of the above will be affected? The answer to that is no. Do you clean out your cupboards of all prescribed medication and over-the-counter remedies? Definitely not! Though, if you look in your cupboard, how many bottles will there be that are almost full, as you tried them and decided they were not right for you?

The above is just to point out the possible dangers we unwittingly incur when we self-medicate without knowing the facts. We are all looking for the elixir of life, and the pharmaceutical and supplement business is an ever-growing market; all are offering benefits and cures for all of our maladies but in taking too much or the wrong combinations we could be doing more harm than good.

Natural hormone creams are available, and many women are finding that these can be helpful not only for menopausal symptoms but for menstrual problems in general.

There are many different supplement 'packages' available, containing a mix of vitamins and minerals or herbal mixes. Pharmacies usually have many different types on sale.

Other forms of alternative therapies, such as flower essences and aromatherapy, have been successfully used for many years, and you do not have to limit yourself to trying just one remedy. Of the English flower essences, the one that is most widely used is known as 'Rescue Remedy' or 'Five Flower Remedy'. It contains the following essences: Star of Bethlehem, rock rose, impatiens, cherry plum and clematis. This combination can be used for a variety of complaints: you may be feeling overwhelmed, or tense and nervous; you may be experiencing anxiety attacks. This remedy can be taken, a few drops at a time, straight from the stock bottle, or drops may be placed in a glass of water or juice. It is surprising how quickly the calming properties kick in.

A mix we have made up for our own use and for friends is one we call 'menopause special'. This contains a mixture of the following essences: walnut, impatiens, olive and scleranthus. Walnut helps with changes in your life. Impatiens more or less says it all. Olive is considered a tonic, and scleranthus is used for mood swings. Please be advised that the base for flower essences is alcohol, so, if you do have dependency problems, be aware that they may not be beneficial for you. You may wish to mix the drops with some cream and rub it into your skin, or you can buy Rescue Remedy as an ointment.

Aromatherapy, like the flower essences, can be used in many ways. Aromatherapy oils are frequently combined with a carrier oil and either massaged into the skin or a few drops added to your bathwater. Clary sage, geranium or lemon placed on your pillow could prove helpful in coping with hot flushes and aid sleep, and sage or cardamom is recommended for irritability. Why not try an aromatherapy massage and experience the wonderful aromas of the different oils being massaged into your skin? An aromatherapist will select the essential oils appropriate to your symptoms. Oils can help with anxiety, insomnia and other negative psychological symptoms as well as general well-being, and the oils can complement any existing regime: conventional or alternative. Again, there are contraindications when using some of the oils, so be responsible and do consult a professional who can advise and treat you.

Health and Well-being

Menstruation can be 'all over the place' during this phase in your life, and your periods may be more frequent or sporadic; there could be spotting between periods, and sometimes you will have a heavy bleed with blood clots. Periods may last longer than you are used to, or you may have a light bleed of a couple of days' duration. All of these can be considered normal, but, if you are at all worried, consult your doctor. It is also handy to mark down on a calendar or in your diary the start date of your period, as this is a question that is always asked when paying a visit to the doctor. Finally, if you have any kind of bleeding from the vagina after menopause, make and *keep* the appointment with your doctor.

Osteoporosis also rears its head as we age, and women start

to lose calcium from their bones at around 35 years of age; again, this can be blamed on the change of our hormones, as it is frequently seen in post-menopausal women. Why, you might wonder? Our bones are living, growing tissue and are constantly changing; our body is constantly breaking down the old bone and replacing it with new. Bones are mainly made up of collagen and calcium phosphate. Formation (done by osteoblasts) is the mechanism of making the bone, and resorption (by osteoclasts) is the breakdown of our bones; these two have to be in balance with each other, and this mechanism is controlled by the hormone oestrogen. When you reach menopause, oestrogen, which is produced in the ovaries, is greatly reduced, and this affects the mechanism. The imbalance causes osteoporosis (porous, fragile and weak bones). If you enter the peri-menopause at an early age or are going though premature menopause, for whatever reason, then you will most likely start to lose the bone mass early as well.

Osteoporosis is a progressive and crippling disease due to the bones becoming weaker as we age and which first presents with the development of osteopenia (thinning of the bones), making your bones fragile and brittle. The most common places you may break a bone are the hips, the spine and above the wrist. A broken hip can limit mobility and lead to loss of independence, while a spine (vertebra) fracture may affect your height and posture.

This disease usually develops over many years and can be relatively painless until you break a bone. Ageing, physical inactivity, poor nutrition, smoking and genetics are major risk factors of osteoporosis; as osteoporosis is also an inherited disease, early detection and taking preventative measures can help slow down its progression. Ask your physician for help and advice on the best course of action for you.

The calcium intake in your diet is important; too little calcium means that you will rob your bones of important minerals that are needed for your bones to stay strong. Dairy products, such as milk, low-fat yoghurt and cheese, green vegetables, tofu, soy products and nuts such as almonds are all rich in calcium.

Below are some indications on how much calcium you require:

Children	800 mg/day
Adolescents	1200 mg/day
Women under 40 years	1000 mg/day
Women over 40 years	1500 mg/day
Men under 60 years	1000 mg/day
Women and men over 60 years	1200 mg/day
Pregnant and nursing women	1200 mg/day

Vitamin D is also important and essential for absorbing calcium. Our main source of Vitamin D is sunlight, but it can also be found in herrings, salmon, sardines, tuna, eggs, milk and other dairy products.

- Did you know that osteoporosis affects women in their thirties and forties as well as the elderly?

- Did you know that a woman's risk of breaking a hip due to osteoporosis is greater than her risks of getting cancer of the breast, cervix, uterus and ovaries combined?

- Did you know that women are 80% more likely to develop osteoporosis than men?

- Did you know that white and Asian women are more likely to suffer from osteoporosis than black women?

- Did you know that Asian women have a higher risk of osteoporosis than Caucasian women?

- Did you know that slender women have less bone mass than heavy or obese women? (Probably because adipose, or fatty, tissue is capable of synthesising oestrogen.)

- Did you know that anorexia nervosa or bulimia creates a higher risk of lower bone density?
- Did you know that one-fourth of white women over 60 years of age have some degree of osteoporosis?

The same can be said for heart disease and strokes; we are more protected during our fertile years than men, but post-menopause we are on a par with men. Worldwide, heart disease is the leading cause of death in men and women; in the UK and Europe, one woman will die from heart disease every six minutes, and in the USA it is one woman every minute. It is not uncommon for women who are experiencing heart problems to be fobbed off with medicine for indigestion. Or, of course, we are stressed and therefore ignore the chest pains – it is just an anxiety attack, we tell ourselves. A lot of the time, women do not seek medical help, as they do not think they are at risk from heart disease. As women gain more information about and become aware of possible health issues that can be directly related to the menopause, they will, hopefully, receive the correct diagnosis and treatment before the problem becomes acute.

Yes, we know you have heard it all before, but don't forget: complacency kills. It makes sense that we should take care of ourselves, and, even if you haven't been interested in your health and well-being in the past, it is never too late to start. If you can't cut out the booze and 'ciggies', cut down, and eating a varied diet that includes fresh fruits and vegetables, proteins and complex carbohydrates in reasonable amounts is a step on the ladder to feeling and becoming healthier; even junk food is getting healthier. It does not mean that you have to give up all of your favourite, though fattening, foods, and it need not get complicated; meals can be adapted to suit you and your family. It is better to keep your weight at an acceptable level that you can maintain than getting overweight and crash dieting. 'Yo-yo' dieting is not good for your body, and, though we are not qualified nutritionists, we could write another book on diet and fitness and it would be one of many on the shelves. Every magazine, newspaper and television programme features items on diets and exercise regimes – it is big business. Sadly, we can become overly concerned with our weight, and it is common nowadays to find middle-aged women who are anorexic and bulimic among the teenage victims of these eating disorders.

We need to keep ourselves fit and healthy, and we will reap the benefits as we get older. The ball, as they say, is in your court. Help and information is widely available on different exercise regimes, and, whether you opt for classes or are motivated enough to get yourself moving, '*moving*' is the key word. Keeping fit need not cost money, and brisk walks and swimming are fairly safe and good ways to get into the swing of things. You may have heard about the 10,000 steps a day programme; all you need is a pedometer and a decent pair of shoes or trainers. Most people walk about 3,000 steps per day; by gradually increasing the amount of walking you do on a daily basis, you will reap the benefits in terms of fitness and stamina. There are many articles and web sites about the 10,000 steps programme; some will even put you in touch with other like-minded people in your area. Not only will you shape up, you will have the opportunity to make new acquaintances. Keeping fit may not lengthen your lifespan, but it will improve your quality of life – if you are healthy in old age, you will reap the benefits.

When you are really motivated, you can progress to strength or resistance training, which will help lower your risk for osteoporosis, as well as aerobics, which helps protect against heart disease and diabetes. Don't underestimate what you are able to do; fitness is not just for the young Adonis (though checking one out will increase the heart rate!). Keeping fit can help alleviate stress, anxiety and insomnia and help keep you regular; what more can you ask for?

Prior to, during and after exercise, it is essential that you do not become dehydrated; we know that fluid intake on a daily basis should be the equivalent of eight glasses of water per day. Depending on your keep-fit routine, it is important to rehydrate the body and, if you exercise regularly, you may need to include an electrolyte supplement drink. Electrolytes – potassium, magnesium and sodium – assist the intestine in absorbing fluids as well as enhancing fluid retention within the body. Although exercise can inhibit hunger, taking in some form of carbohydrate within three hours after exercise will help stop depletion of muscle tissue. During exercise, the body uses carbohydrates and proteins as fuel and carries on fuelling the body after exercise has finished; if you are strength training, you are, in theory, building muscle, but if you are not eating properly, you may be depleting the muscle you are trying to build. That's why any form of diet and exercise should be monitored and understood in order for you and your body to reap the benefits.

It is all right giving out the advice, but what do *we* do? Well, we are both fairly active on a daily basis, even though we could and should do more; like most, we suffer from a case of 'I'll start tomorrow'. We *do* have reasonably healthy diets, as well as watching our weight – or, more truthfully, the numbers that appear on the scales. One of us smokes and the other likes a regular tipple; we both have cellulite and KY can be found in our shopping trolley, so we are on the 'normal' list and not super women. Exercising can be sporadic, but we have taken classes in yoga and tai chi, and we are currently learning to horse ride – tally ho girls! – and play golf, and kickboxing could be next on the list. As we both have dogs and pedometers, it is not too hard to reach 10,000 steps most days.

Smoking: what can we say? We all know the detrimental effects of smoking, but consider the incidence of smoking-related diseases, including lung cancer, mouth and throat cancers, strokes, heart failure, bronchitis and emphysema; of course, any of these ailments will shorten your lifespan.

Passive smokers – a non-smoker inhaling the smoke from cigarettes – have as many smoke-related problems as smokers do. That is why many countries prohibit smoking in public places, especially work environments.

There is no safe limit when it comes to smoking cigarettes, and it has been proven that the nicotine in cigarettes is addictive and has a negative impact on day-to-day memory. Most smokers realise that it is difficult to quit, but it is not impossible; if you want to quit due to health problems *or* you would like to put your money to better use, go see your doctor and let them help you to take this step.

Post-Menopause

Phew! At last, post-menopause: this is when most of the menopausal symptoms have decreased and you have stopped menstruating. You can now take time to reflect on this part of your life. Some women mourn the passing of their fertility, as, in theory,[3] this is the end of the childbearing years; you are moving on from a large and important phase in life, and you can feel emotionally 'lost'.

Parenthood may have been, until now, your primary role. It is OK to feel sad and reflect on this time, because this is how you come to terms with who you were and what that meant to you and others close to you, and, importantly, where the future will take you. The maternal void you may feel when the kids leave home is also known as the 'empty nest syndrome'. Don't forget, your partner may be feeling the same sense of loss, especially if they have enjoyed a close relationship with the children; a house that has always been filled with the noise of 'family' may now seem eerily

---

[3] Due to the advances in fertility treatment, women who are healthy and still have a womb but have finished menstruating may be able to carry a child by having a donated egg fertilised and transplanted into the womb.

quiet. For some, it will be filled in the role of being a grandparent, and that brings just as much pleasure and heartache as it did with your own children – but what a joy they are!

For many couples, the role of parenting is ongoing, due to the responsibility of 'parenting' parents, and this can be emotionally and physically draining for all concerned. Coming to terms with this role reversal is not easy; we always want our parents to be just that – Mum and Dad – and home carers are, so often, forgotten. It is vital that you seek and take any help that is offered, because stress, anxiety and depression can so easily spiral out of control, leaving you feeling resentful towards parents who so often bear no resemblance to those who raised you. Sadly, it is becoming commonplace for the elderly to be victimised and abused by their families. It's heavy stuff being an adult.

But, if you now have the opportunity to pursue the things you wanted to try but never had the time for, this can be the time in your life when you change direction, especially career-wise. To coin a phrase, you will never be too old to try something for the first time; even if you find it is not what you want, you had a go. Your capacity for learning doesn't stop just because your hormone levels have dropped – your brain is still eager and hungry for new input. Don't just dip your toe in the water; take the plunge and go for it, girl! The fertility body clock has stopped, but the 'life' clock is still ticking, and not in a favourable direction – time isn't on your side!

★ SMILE TIME ★

My Younger Days

When I was in my younger days,
I weighed a few pounds less,
I needn't hold my tummy in
To wear a belted dress.

But now that I am older,
I've set my body free;
There's comfort of elastic
Where once my waist would be.

Inventor of those high-heeled shoes,
My feet have not forgiven;
I have to wear a nine now,
But used to wear a seven.

And how about those pantyhose?
They're sized by weight, you see,
So how come when I put them on
The crotch is at my knees?

I need to wear these glasses
As the prints were getting smaller;
And it wasn't very long ago
I know that I was taller.

Though my hair has turned to grey
And my skin no longer fits,
On the inside, I'm still the same old me,
Just the outside's changed a bit.

Maya Angelou

A lot of women find they have become complacent about how they dress and look; it feels like a really big, pointless effort, especially if make-up and hair is ruined when a hot flush strikes. Don't give up on yourself; looking at the mirror and seeing a reflection that looks OK is a morale boost. We know that, over the years, your appearance will have changed and, while some have altered their style, others will feel left in a 'time warp'.

So, if you have been stuck in a rut with your hairstyle, make-up and clothes, grab your daughter or a friend and go shopping. You will be surprised how little it costs to see who is under there, waiting to come out. The larger department shops with cosmetic counters are more than happy to advise on skin creams and cleansing routines and help give you a new look in make-up (don't forget, they are hoping you will buy!). Visit a wig boutique and try out different styles and colours before rushing off to the hairdresser's and making a mistake that you will have to live with for a few weeks. Then, of course, there are all those clothes shops.

Size is irrelevant, so there is no excuse for not throwing caution to the wind and trying on clothes that make a statement of who you are now: a woman, a W-O-M-A-N! Remember, it costs nothing to look, and what a boost it can be for your confidence. Who knows, you may like what you see. The smile that spreads across your face says it all!

Don't forget underwear; nobody looks good with a visible panty line. And your new wardrobe will be pointless if you are still cramming your boobs into a bra with a questionable fit. If you are not sure about your size, try these guidelines: measure underneath your bust, adding four inches if the measurement is an even number and five inches if the measurement is an odd number. Then measure around the fullest part of your bust to give you the cup size. If your measurement is the same as the under-bust measurement, then you will need an 'A' cup.

One inch more = a 'B' cup; two inches more = a 'C' cup, and so on. Still not sure? Don't worry; you will usually find an assistant who is trained and can advise on the right kind of bra – it will make a difference to your figure, and you will have lots of choice. From plain to lacy and in an array of colours from delicate peaches and cream to purples and black, under-wired and padded; you can be voluptuous or, if you are well endowed, you can minimise.

Even, at the end of the day, if all you have bought is coffee and lunch, you will go back home feeling great and ready for the next excursion, when, we are sure, you will be ready to invest in the updated you!.

If post-menopause can now account for a third of our lives, we have the chance of new beginnings, and, whatever they may be, as they say, there is always a light at the end of the tunnel, and now you have found it.

At one time, a woman who had gone through the meno-pause was considered to be a wise woman; she had the wisdom of her age, of 'knowing a lifetime', and she was revered, a matriarch. So hold your head high and face the future: you are a woman of your time.

★ SMILE TIME ★

The Purple Hat

Age 3:   She looks at herself and sees a Queen.

Age 8:   She looks at herself and sees Cinderella.

Age 15:   She looks at herself and sees an Ugly Sister (Mum, I can't go to school looking like this!).

Age 20:   She looks at herself and sees 'too fat/too thin, too short/too tall, too straight/too curly' – but decides she's going out anyway.

Age 30:   She looks at herself and sees 'too fat/too thin, too short/too tall, too straight/too curly' – but decides she doesn't have time to fix it, so she's going out anyway.

Age 40:   She looks at herself and sees 'clean' and goes out anyway.

Age 50:   She looks at herself and sees 'I am' and goes wherever she wants to go.

Age 60:   She looks at herself and reminds herself of all the people who can't even see themselves in the mirror any more. Goes out and conquers the world.

Age 70:   She looks at herself and sees wisdom, laughter and ability, goes out and enjoys life.

Age 80:   Doesn't bother to look. Just puts on a purple hat and goes out to have fun with the world.

Men – Oh Please!

Yes, girls, men have been with us throughout this chapter, menstruation, menopause and hysterectomy; it is only fair we give them a mention. Seriously, the male 'menopause' was debated for a long time before it became accepted, a bit like female sexual dysfunction.

Is a man middle-aged when he is 40? Personally, we both think that a man approaches middle age when turning 50. But, if you take into consideration the lifespan of men and women, women do usually live longer. Men should be considered middle-aged at 40. Right, girls, now we have a good excuse for marrying a younger man, since we women live longer.

Men do go through a *'men*-opause' or, more correctly, andropause (decreased testosterone levels associated with the normal ageing processes), just like women do. After the age of 40, fertility can decline by as much as 70%, and, because a lot of couples are delaying starting a family, men are now just as likely to have fertility problems. According to an article in the *Daily Mail* (Tuesday, 6 June 2006), 'Other factors thought to be responsible for declining male fertility include being overweight, smoking, excessive amounts of alcohol or coffee, too much soy, traffic pollution, cannabis, using a laptop, and traces of the female pill that have passed into our water supply.' Now there's food for thought.

Did you know that many of the symptoms for men are similar to the ones we experience?

So look out for these, girls:

- lower sex drive

- not as energetic

- lack of stamina

- life holds no joy

- grumpy, negative outlook

- 'softer' erections

- decreased sports prowess

- more after-dinner naps

- less enthusiastic about work

- suffers bouts of depression.[4]

Wow, looking at this list, we both think some men go through 'men-opause' at a very early age – especially considering 'more after-dinner naps'.

Do men suffer? Yes, we believe they do, and very much so. Most of the symptoms are a decrease or reduction in qualities that a man associates with being a man. We learn to come to terms with our loss of fertility; does the same apply to your man?

Do men talk openly about their 'change' with each other, their partner or their doctor? We don't think they do. Sometimes, we all need a sympathetic ear and a shoulder to cry on; if you and your man are not able to communicate about these changes, try leaving relevant information around for him to see. Men can seek help, as long as they know where to look or whom to ask.

Let's face it: a household with a menopausal woman and a

---

[4] From www.consumerhealthdigest.

'men-opausal' man must be like living in a war zone. Where does that leave your relationship or any family member who is stuck in the middle?

Testosterone treatment is available for men, though it poses similar risks as HRT does for women. The doctor would need to look at the family history and lifestyle of your man before possible treatment could commence; testosterone therapy would not be given if there is an instance of breast or prostate cancer. Liver, heart and kidney disease and diabetes mellitus also pose a problem, as well as some conventional medication, e.g. blood thinners.

A questionnaire survey of 1,885 men aged 55, 65 and 75 years of age has been carried out in Linkoping, Sweden, regarding hot flushes in men, which are not related to exercise or a warm environment. 1,381 were eligible for evaluation (33 others were analysed separately, as the men had been castrated).

- Hot flushes of any frequency were experienced by 33.1%

- 4.3% experienced hot flushes a few times per week

- 1.3% experienced hot flushes daily.

Half of the men experiencing hot flushes were bothered by them, and a relationship was found between hot flushes and other symptoms thought to be related to low testosterone, though no further studies regarding testosterone replacement were carried out.[5]

Although osteoporosis is seen as a woman's disease, men are affected, but not to the same extent as women; as men have larger skeletons, the bone loss is slower. They tend to have a shorter lifespan, and, of course, they don't have the rapid hormonal changes of oestrogen as we women do; these are

---

[5] Spetz, A C, M G Fredriksson and M L Hammar, University Hospital, Linkoping, Sweden.

some of the reasons why we do not see as many men with osteoporosis.

If he is reluctant to take your word for his 'mood swings', get him to log on to www.andropause.com and www.menstuff.org for more information relating to these topics. Men, remember: the 'change' is not an illness; it is just a natural process in your life. We wish we could stop the clock for you, but we can't.

Points to ponder: did you know that Viagra is one of the top-selling medications purchased via the Internet? And (our personal favourite), while surfing the Internet, we came across an article by a Nicholas Bakalar, and it relates to a study carried out at Brookfield Zoo, in Chicago, about menopausal female gorillas. Yes, we are serious! It states, 'They may not have hot flushes or experience drastic mood swings. But a new study of captive female gorillas suggests that, like human females, the animals go through physiological changes when their reproductive days are ending.' So, if your other half is moaning about your mood swings, ask him to spare a thought for captive male gorillas; they can't take off to the pub or go fishing when her hormones are raging. We imagine them sitting quietly in a corner, hoping not to be noticed by their significant other!

Well, Woman?

In this chapter, we would like to make you more familiar with female diseases and illnesses associated with post-menopause and ageing, as well as what happens on your yearly visit to the gynaecologist or Well Woman Clinic and how to do your monthly self-examination. If you are already familiar with the gynaecologist exam, you can skip these few pages and go directly to the self-examination section; whether you know it or not, it is always good to refresh your memory. Self-examination may make you feel uncomfortable, but, when done on a monthly basis, you learn what your body looks and feels like when it is healthy, and who better to inspect than yourself?

Surprisingly, many women who have an active sex life or have had children are still in the dark regarding their own bodies, and, as we age, it is important to have regular health checks, as prevention is better than cure. Well Woman Clinics are usually offered at your local GP practice, hospitals and private clinics. Usually, a 'well woman' check includes taking a swab from the neck of the cervix – a cervical smear, or you may know them as Pap smears. As well as an internal examination, you will be given a breast examination. Samples of urine and blood are taken, and your blood pressure and weight are checked. This is also a good time to ask any questions you may have regarding your health. You should have a routine gynaecological exam yearly, and a mammogram and bone density exam every two years after turning 40 and yearly after 50, though you may have to pay for the mammogram and bone density exam unless you are known to be at risk of osteoporosis or breast problems.

The yearly 'gyno' check makes a lot of women feel a little

uptight, especially if it is the first time. When you book your appointment, you will be asked the date of your last menstruation; obviously, it makes sense not to have the exam done while you are menstruating, and it is more comfortable, breastwise, seven to ten days after your last menses; post-menopause, this is not an issue. If you have any questions to ask, now is a good time to sit down and make the list. Be honest when making the list, and don't withhold any information from your doctor because you feel embarrassed; they are professionals and have, no doubt, seen and heard it all before.

If sexually active, it is best not to have sex the day before the exam, and do not take any yeast medications, use spermicides or douche for twenty-four hours beforehand, as it could interfere with the Pap smear test and results. When you arrive, ask the nurse if they need a urine sample, which is usual. They will also tell you how to collect the sample: you will need to part the labia, the lip-like part of your vulva, pass a little urine into the toilet and then urinate into the test bottle mid-stream, before you finish urinating; this is called a mid-stream urine sample. It is not as messy as it sounds, and you can get quite adept at peeing into a bottle! Also, having an empty bladder makes for a more comfortable exam.

More often than not, you will be seen by the doctor or health care professional (to save repeating, we will use 'doctor') prior to your internal exam and you will have your blood pressure, pulse rate, temperature and weight checked. Your doctor will ask relevant questions and discuss your health in general; we hope you haven't forgotten your list, because now you will have the chance to raise any questions that you might have. You will probably know your doctor from previous visits, but remember that you should not have a physical examination from anyone you do not feel comfortable with and there should always be a second person present during an examination; this is standard practice and protects both you and your doctor.

You will usually be shown into an examination room, where you will be asked to undress, including removing underwear, and, though taking off all of your clothes may feel strange, it is necessary. You will be asked to put on a gown and to sit on the exam table; usually there is a cover that you can have over you. You will be given a few minutes to change, and the doctor will knock and ask if you are ready before entering the room. Regardless of your doctor being male or female, they understand your apprehension prior to these exams, and we have always found them to be patient and totally professional.

An examination is carried out with you in a sitting position as well as lying down; you will have the sheet or gown covering you, and the doctor will only uncover the parts of your body being examined. Usually, the breasts are checked first; you will be sitting up at this point, as they will look at the shape of the breast and ask you to raise your arms above your head, feeling for any changes in your underarm. The breast exam may continue with you lying down. The doctor will examine each breast by pressing all around the breast area, starting from the outside and working toward the nipple area. This is not uncomfortable. If you do not know how to examine your breasts, the doctor will show you and tell you what you should be feeling for. If you have any history of breast problems, you may also be given a mammogram or an ultrasound, sometimes both; early detection can lead to a positive outcome.

Next, the pelvic exam; it is not anyone's favourite part of the appointment, but, for the sake of good health… You will be asked to lie down, keep your breathing nice and relaxed, count the dots in the tiles on the ceiling, make small talk – do whatever it takes to keep you relaxed. You may be asked to rest your feet in stirrups. These are metal triangular loops at the bottom of the bed. They may look a little scary, but they are just there to rest your legs in and are not uncomfortable.

Otherwise, you will be asked to draw your feet together and let your knees relax to the sides; we all feel a little vulnerable, legs akimbo, but is only for a short time. The doctor will put on gloves and examine the outside of your vagina, the vulva area, to make sure there are no sores, ingrown hair, blocked glands, herpes blisters or unusual swelling. Next, the doctor will want to look at the inside of your vagina and will do so with the help of a speculum. A speculum is a thin piece of plastic or metal, with a hinge on one end that allows it to open and close. The doctor will warm the speculum and tell you when they are about to place the speculum inside you so it doesn't come as a shock.

Once the speculum is in the vagina, it can be opened to allow the doctor to see inside. Putting in and opening the speculum should not be painful, although some women say that it can cause a bit of pressure and discomfort. Naturally, if this is your first exam, you might feel a little tense. Because the vagina is surrounded by muscles that can contract or relax, the exam can be more comfortable if you try to stay calm and relax the muscles in that area. Count those dots on the ceiling again! After the speculum is in place, the doctor will shine a light inside the vagina to look for anything unusual, such as redness, swelling, discharge or sores. They will then do a Pap smear, which involves a little scraping of the cervix to pick up cells from that area. It does not hurt but might feel strange. The good news is that this part of the exam is over quickly. It is not unusual afterwards to have a little spotting of blood from the vagina, but inform the doctor if it's more than a few drops. The cells that have been collected are sent to a laboratory, where they are studied for any abnormalities that may indicate infection or warning signs of cervical cancer.

Because the ovaries and uterus are so far inside a woman's body that they can't be seen at all, even with the speculum inserted and open, the doctor will need to feel them to be sure they are healthy. While your legs are still in the stirrups, and after the speculum is removed from the vagina, the doctor will put lubricant on two fingers (of course, gloves are still on) and slide the fingers inside your vagina. Using the other hand, they will press on the outside of your lower abdomen (the area between your vagina and your stomach). With two hands, one on the outside and one on the inside, the doctor can make sure that the ovaries and uterus are the right size and free of cysts or other growths. During this part of the exam, you may feel a little pressure or discomfort. Again, it is important to relax your muscles and take slow, deep breaths if you feel nervous. In some clinics, ultrasound machines are available to do this particular exam.

Finally, a rectal exam. That's right! If your doctor doesn't make this exam regular practice, ask for it. It may sound strange to actually request this, but it is important. This step, in which one finger is in the vagina and the other is in the rectum, helps detect rectal lesions and growths (an early sign of colon cancer) and also helps point out endometriosis, ovarian cysts, and the alignment of the uterus and other pelvic organs. Since you are already on the exam table, let the doctor do it so it is over and done with in one go and you don't have to go back for one more exam.

At last, the physical part of the exam is over, and it only took about three to five minutes. Your own doctor may do the exam in a different order, but it will probably include all of the above.

Afterward, you'll be left alone to get dressed; ask for a couple of tissues to wipe away the excess lubricant and if you bleed a little, ask the nurse for a panty-liner to protect your underwear. Remember, only a few drops is normal – nothing like a menstruation. Now the final step: back into the doctor's office. If you haven't discussed your questions or forgot to ask something, now's the time. Again, don't be afraid of asking questions that sound stupid or silly; there is no such thing as a stupid question about your body, and this is the best time to get professional answers for your questions. You may be asked to make another appointment for between seven and ten days later for the results of your Pap smear; if not, the doctor will usually contact you with the results. If the physical exam left you not wanting another, remember that each time it gets easier and it really is necessary to be a 'well woman'.

As a matter of interest:

While writing this book, we have become more aware of our own bodies and the importance of having well-woman check-ups. As mentioned, cervical cancer is treatable if it is diagnosed early, and, with this in mind, we conducted a 'quickie' poll.

This was conducted at the stables where we go riding, and we were making the most of the mainly middle-aged women whom we see there.

This is what we asked for:

- Age

- Nationality

- Do you have a regular gynaecological check-up?

- If the answer is yes, how often and when were you last tested?

- If no, can you give a reason for not having the test done? Please be honest with your reply.

17 ladies completed the form, with the ages ranging from 25 to 58 years. The nationalities were: British (5), British/Bahraini (1), Irish (3), Swedish (1), Australian (1), South African (1), Canadian (1), American (2), Dutch (1), Polish (1).

14 of the 17 ladies had regular gynaecological check-ups, including a Pap test, with time spans ranging from six months to two years.

The three ladies who did not have regular testing gave the following reasons:

- too lazy – never enough time;
- can't stand doctors, especially male gynaecologists, and female ones are hard to find.

The third lady had just had her first one done at the age of 27, and the reason given for not having had a Pap previously was: 'Nerves! But I am aware how important it is and will continue to get checked regularly. (And for others who are nervous, I assure you there's nothing to worry about!).'

We were pleased to find that most of the ladies we spoke to were aware for the need of regular testing and knew that being post-menopause did not mean they were less vulnerable, but having a regular gyno check-up was not on their list of favourite things to do.

Mammogram

There is a lot of confusion about when and how often to have a mammogram. Today, the recommendation is that women over 40 should have a mammogram every two years, and women who are 50 and above every year, unless you are considered to be at risk from breast cancer, in which case you should be under the care of your doctor. Film screen mammography involves minimal radiation exposure – even less than an ordinary X-ray – so do not worry about excess radiation.

A mammogram can be arranged through your doctor or Well Woman Clinic or privately; many clinics and private hospitals offer a 'Well Woman Package', which can include blood and urine analysis, measuring cholesterol levels and hormone levels, Pap smear, gynaecological examination, mammogram and/or ultrasound as well as a follow-up appointment.

When you arrive at the X-ray department, you will be seen by a radiologist, who will want to know if you have had previous mammograms or procedures on your breasts, including breast implants. If you have had surgery, such as a benign biopsy or surgery to reduce the size of your breasts, the radiologist will want to know where those scars are in case the scar tissue has to be distinguished from another kind of breast abnormality. If you've had breast cancer surgery, small metal balls will be taped onto your skin to mark your scar. Your scar defines the site with the highest risk of recurrence.

You will be shown into the X-ray room and you will be asked to remove upper-body clothing, e.g. shirt and bra, though you are given an examination gown. Don't know why, but it always feels cold in these rooms, so be prepared. You will also be asked if you have used talcum powder or deodorant, as using these prior to a mammogram can give a false image; talc is calcium-based and it will show up as deposits in the breast. The X-ray machine consists of two plates; one breast at a time is placed and positioned on the lower plate, while the upper plate compresses the breast. Your arms may be hanging down by the side of your body, or you may be asked to hold onto two handles located above the X-ray machine. The X-ray itself is as quick as taking a photograph, but the radiologist will check each plate before proceeding; this is to make sure the X-ray has been taken. Each breast has two images taken: one, as described above, and a second with the plates placed on either side of the breast, in profile. For most women mammography is not painful – just causes a little discomfort – but, if it is too painful, do not hesitate to tell the radiologist so they can reduce the compression. Compression of the breast is necessary to reduce the thickness of the breast, as the X-ray beam should penetrate as few layers of overlapping tissues as possible in order to get a more accurate reading.

At least one radiologist, a doctor specialising in imaging the body, reads the mammogram. Having two radiologists read your mammogram reduces the chance of missing a problem by about 10–15%. Your doctor then examines each area and decides if it needs further evaluation, in which case you may be asked to have an additional mammogram or a breast ultra-sound examination.

Some women will have both a mammogram and an ultra-sound. An ultrasound can provide more information about the health of your breasts, and it is most commonly used on women who have had breast implants or prostheses, those who have dense breasts – breasts with a high proportion of fibro-glandular tissue, usually younger women – or when a suspicious area shows up on the mammogram. A breast ultrasound takes about twenty to thirty minutes and, as with the mammogram, you will need to remove your clothes. An ultrasound is a painless procedure. A doctor or sonographer will apply a gel to the breast area (if you have had an ultra-sound during pregnancy, it is the same procedure). The gel is used so that the sound waves can 'see' through the skin to the breast tissue. The sound waves form a picture on the monitor and any irregularities can be seen.

In some clinics, you will see the doctor after the X-rays/ultrasound have been completed or you will be given an appointment to return to the clinic, otherwise your results will be sent to your own doctor and you will need to make an appointment at your surgery. A lot of us expect the results to be bad news; most of us will have felt 'lumpy' breasts at some point, so do make your concerns known and, if you have any questions, ask away; don't spend sleepless nights wondering 'What if…?' Abnormal findings do not necessarily mean cancer.

There is also digital mammography, which uses the same technique as film screen mammography, but the image is recorded directly into a computer. The image can then be enlarged or highlighted. If there is a suspicious area, your doctors can use the computer to take a closer look. Right now, what doctors can see with digital mammography is not quite as clear as what they can see with film, and the technique is more expensive and not as widely available. But, in the future, digital mammography will be more common. Your radiologist may read your mammogram with the help of computer-aided detection (CAD) programs, and then send your mammogram to you and your doctor via the Internet.

- Women in the UK aged 50 and above can have a mammogram every three years on the NHS.

- Private 'Well Woman Packages' can be adapted to suit your needs, including bone density scan, pelvic scan and, of course, whatever you can afford. Yes, health care and preventative measures come at a price.

- If you have breast implants, the mammogram may need to be adapted to show as much breast tissue as possible. Compression of the breasts will not damage your implants, but, if you think there is a problem with the implants, mention this before having the mammogram.

- If you are still menstruating, you should wait until at least ten days after your last menstruation before having a mammogram; the breasts will be less tender.

★ SMILE TIME ★

Ode to a Mammogram

For years and years they told me,
Be careful of your breasts.
Don't ever squeeze or bruise them,
And give them monthly tests.
So I heeded all their warnings,
And protected them by law.
Watched them very carefully,
And always wore my bra.

After thirty years of astute care,
My gyno, Dr Pruitt,
Said I should get a mammogram.
'OK,' I said, 'let's do it.'
'Stand up here real close,' she said,
(She got my boob in line),
'And tell me when it hurts,' she said,
'Ah, yes! Right there, that's fine.'
She stepped upon a pedal,
I could not believe my eyes!
A plastic plate came slamming down,
My hooter's in a vice!
My skin was stretched and mangled,
From underneath my chin.
My poor boob was being squashed,
To Swedish Pancake thin.
Excruciating pain I felt,
Within its vice-like grip.
A prisoner in this vicious thing,
My poor defenceless tit!
'Take a deep breath,' she said to me,
Who does she think she's kidding?
My chest is mashed in her machine,
And woozy I am getting.
'There, that's good,' I heard her say.
(The room was slowly swaying.)
'Now, let's have the other one.'
Have mercy, I was praying.
It squeezed me from both up and down,
It squeezed me from both sides.
I'll bet *she's* never had this done,
To *her* soft little hide.
Next time that they make me do this,
I will request a blindfold.
I have no wish to see again,

My knockers getting steamrolled.
If I had no problem when I came in,
I surely have one now.
If there had been a cyst in there,
It would have gone 'ker-pow!'
This machine was created by a man,
Of this, I have no doubt.
I'd like to stick his balls in there,
And see how *they* come out!

Author unknown

Monthly Self-Exam

A monthly self-exam will take no more than ten minutes of your time, and learning what your body looks and feels like when it is healthy will make it easier to notice any changes. If an apple a day keeps the doctor away, then ten minutes a month will help keep disease at bay.

BREAST SELF-EXAM

If you are still menstruating, examine the breast a few days after your period ends. You will need to stand in front of a mirror, so we guess you will either be in the bathroom or bedroom. Before we begin, why not take a good look at your naked body? It's beautiful! Be comfortable in your skin; look all around your body – this is you. Celebrate you and learn to love your body; do not be embarrassed or feel disgust. Look at yourself in the mirror and smile; guaranteed 'she' will smile back! OK, that's enough; down to business.

1. Stand facing the mirror with your arms by your side and take the time to look at your breasts; they should be evenly shaped (though it is usual to have one breast slightly larger than the other – usually the left breast) without any visible distortions or swelling.

Look for any of the following: dimpling, puckering or bulging of the skin; an inverted nipple: the nipple is pushed inwards; sore skin, a rash, redness or swelling. If you find any of these, seek medical advice.

2. Now, raise your arms and look for the same changes. While you're at the mirror, gently roll each nipple between your finger and thumb and check for nipple discharge; this could be a milky or yellow fluid, which is not unusual, or blood, which is not OK – see your doctor.

3. Finally, examine your breasts while lying down; your head is on a pillow, and a folded towel should be placed under the left shoulder, as this helps to spread the breast tissue. Place the left hand at the back of your head, leaving the area of the left breast and armpit open and accessible. With your right hand flat with fingers together, feel around the breast from your collarbone to the top of your abdomen and from your armpit to your cleavage, using a circular movement. Be firm and cover the whole breast, including the nipple, then check your armpit in the same way. Now repeat with the right breast.

   Many women find that the easiest way to feel their breasts is when their skin is wet and soapy, so they like to do this step in the shower. Examine your entire breast, using the same hand movements as described above.

   If your breast feels lumpy, check the same area of the opposite breast; it may just be your natural shape, but, if you are at all worried, make an appointment with your doctor. It's better to be on the safe side.

What do we really know about our breasts and breast cancer? Most of us would panic and think the worst at finding a lump in the breast, but what about a rash on the outside of the breast? Is this cause for concern? Read on and be informed.

If you notice a rash on your breast, would you put it down to an allergy or a sweat rash? This, of course, may be what it is. But if you have a persistent redness that resembles eczema, possible itching and oozing, and crusting of the nipple and areola area, will you consult your doctor? It is said that nine out of ten women who have these symptoms will have Paget's disease of the breast or DCIS, which is short for 'ductal carcinoma in situ' and refers to cancer in the milk ducts. These symptoms are due to the presence of Paget's cells in the skin of the nipple. Paget's cells are large, irregular cells that are themselves not cancerous but which are almost always associated with a cancer in the breast, and diagnosis and treatment are the same as for tumorous breast cancer.

Paget's disease of the breast is associated with women who have no children or had them later in life, early menstruation, late menopause or a family history of breast cancer. According to information on the breast cancer site,[6] one or two women in every 100 who have breast cancer will have Paget's disease and the age group more commonly (but not exclusively) affected is women in their 50s.

If you notice an unusual rash on your breast, will you wait or will you seek medical advice? When it comes to your health, don't think you are making a fuss about nothing or put off making an appointment until tomorrow (whenever 'tomorrow' might be). Make an appointment, keep the appointment; if you come out of the doctor's with a pre-scription for a topical cream to treat your sweat rash, that's fine, but at least you will have peace of mind.

VULVA EXAMINATION

That's right: a vulva exam, and this is why. Doctors are seeing an increase of infectious diseases, such as herpes and genital warts, plus cancer and precancerous conditions, especially in younger women. Do not be alarmed; be armed with the right

---

[6] www.cancerbackup.org.uk.

information. As with the breast exam, a few minutes once a month is all it takes. If you have had previous treatment for any vulva disease, it is important for you to perform a self-exam regularly.

The vulva refers to a woman's external genital area.

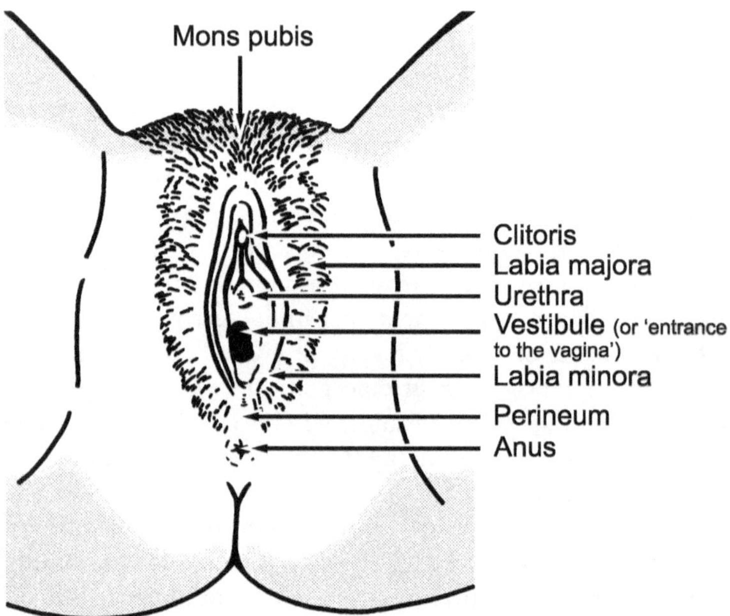

Remember when you had your yearly gyno check-up, the doctor examined your vulva prior to taking a Pap smear. Now the ball is in your court, and every woman over the age of eighteen should do a monthly self-exam, regardless of being sexually active or not. Do not feel embarrassed when doing a vulva exam; a woman's genitalia is inside – not on display, like a man's, for all to see – and we all know how many times he checks his!

For this self-exam, you will need a hand-held mirror. Make sure the room has plenty of light; your eyes are just as important for this exam. Make yourself comfortable, either on the floor or sitting on a chair or the bed, whichever position feels comfortable and allows you to see and examine the vulva area. Check out the diagram and become familiar with the names of the areas you need to examine. Use you free hand to examine the vulva, using your fingers to feel for any lumps or changes in the area. Start from the 'mons pubis' and work your way down to the clitoris, the labia minora, labia majora, the perineum and the anus.

- Look at the vulva in the mirror.

- Look at the colour of the skin; is there any pigmentation or whitening?

- Is there any thickening of the skin, e.g. warts or ulcers?

- Do you have pain, inflammation, sores or constant itching?

As with the breast exam, if you have any concerns, consult with your doctor; early detection, diagnosis and treatment usually equates to a positive outcome.

Get into the habit of monthly self-exams – it's a good habit to have. On a day-to-day basis it is always good to have a look at the colour of your urine – if it is dark in colour you may need to drink more water – and look at the stools you pass – the consistency and colour. You don't need to put your head down the loo, just be aware of your bodily functions.

The Love of Our Life, Again

What can we say? We have to include him; if we don't take notice of their health, who will? Apart from the diseases of the reproductive system, the vulva exam and the yearly gynaecological check-up, the diseases above apply to your man and he can also do the breast self-exam. Men do develop breast cancer so make sure he knows what to look for.

Health centres, clinics and hospitals offer a 'Well Man'

screening, and he will have to drop his trousers for his testicular and prostate check, so, when you make an appointment for yourself, make one for him. In the meantime, these are some of the symptoms associated with prostate and testicular cancer.

PROSTATE SYMPTOMS

- Frequency in urinating, especially at night
- More visits to the toilet, may even wet yourself at times
- Difficulty in starting to urinate; blood in the urine
- Pain or straining or taking a long time to finish
- A weak flow and the feeling that your bladder has not emptied
- Pain on ejaculating; difficulty in getting an erection
- Pain in the genital area
- Pain in the lower back, hips or pelvis.

SELF-EXAMINATION OF TESTICLES

As with the breast exam, a monthly examination of the testicles is a good habit to get into, and a good time for this exam is after a shower or bath, when the scrotal skin is warm and relaxed.

- Hold the scrotum in the palm of your hands; it is usual to have one testicle larger than the other or one that hangs slightly lower down.
- Note the size and weight of the testicles and feel each testicle in turn.
- You should feel a soft tube at the top and back of the testicle. This is the epididymis, which carries and stores sperm.
- You should also be able to feel the firm, smooth tube of the spermatic cord, which runs up from the epididymis.

- Feel the testicle itself. It should be smooth, with no lumps or swellings.

It is unusual to develop cancer in both testicles at the same time; if one testicle feels lumpy, compare it with the other. If he does find a lump, just remember that, as with breasts, not all lumps are malignant. If he is experiencing any problems and is reluctant to go to the doctor's, make the appointment and nag him into submission!

Gynaecological Cancer

The most common female reproductive cancers are cervical, ovarian and uterine, and, if you are experiencing any of the following, you need to see the doctor. Women at all ages can be affected, but these cancers are more frequently seen in women who are aged 45 to 65 (pre- and post-menopausal).

- Unusual vaginal bleeding or discharge, especially if you are post-menopause

- A sore that does not heal

- Pain or pressure in the pelvic area

- A persistent change in bowel or bladder habits

- Frequent indigestion or abdominal bloating

- A thickening or lump that causes pain or can be seen or felt.

OVARIAN TUMOURS

Older women appear to be more susceptible to ovarian cancer, with more than half of the deaths occurring in women between 55 and 74 years of age while approximately one-quarter of ovarian cancer deaths occur in women between 35 and 54 years of age.

However, the more children a woman has, the lower her risk of ovarian cancer. Early age at first pregnancy, older ages of final pregnancy and the use of low-dose oral contraceptive pills have also been shown to have a protective effect, and ovarian cancer is reduced in women after tubal ligation (sterilisation).

Few symptoms present until the tumour has grown to a relatively big size, and the symptoms can include abdominal discomfort and pain, digestive upset and, later, more severe pain, anaemia and a hard mass that can be felt. This is a solid tumour in the ovary, which may be either benign (not cancerous) or malignant (cancerous). Also, you may notice a deepening of the voice and hair growth; if you are experiencing any of the above symptoms, however vague, seek medical advice.

Treatment involves surgery to remove the tumour or, usually, the ovary and fallopian tube. In some cases of malignancy, a hysterectomy may be required. Chemotherapy and/or radiotherapy are likely to be needed if the tumour is cancerous. It is not known what causes ovarian cancers, and the outcome may be fatal if the cancer spreads to other parts of the body and secondary growths occur.

UTERINE CANCER

Symptoms of uterine cancer include abnormal bleeding – bleeding that is not connected with menstruation. In post-menopausal women, this may be in the form of a watery or mucus-like discharge that may be streaked in with blood.

Cancer of the uterus is a growth of malignant cells in the uterus or womb and is a relatively common form of cancer in women. Once again, it is most common in older women past the menopause, especially between the ages 50 to 60.

Treatment involves surgery to remove the uterus (hysterectomy) and usually the ovaries and fallopian tubes. Radiotherapy and treatment with progesterone may be necessary. The outlook is quite good for the majority of women who have not waited to seek diagnosis and treatment; otherwise, there is a risk that the cancer will spread to set up secondary growths elsewhere, which are likely to be fatal.

Again, the cause is unknown, but the risk of developing cancer in the uterus increases with diabetes mellitus, a family history of breast or ovarian cancer, a menstrual cycle in which an egg is not released and therefore there is no input of progesterone, and oestrogen therapy. Women who are overweight and those who have high blood pressure or hormonal imbalances are also at risk.

CERVICAL CANCER

Cervical cancer is cancer of the 'neck', or cervix, of the womb, and is one of the most successfully treated cancers when detected in the early or even precancerous stage. Though the UK has one of the lowest rates of infection from HPV (human papillomavirus) in Europe out of the 3,000 cases diagnosed yearly there will still be 1,000 deaths, and cervical cancer is rife in developing countries. In the precancerous stage, readily detectable changes occur in the cells lining the surface of the cervix. These can be identified by means of a cervical smear test (Pap smear). As we have said, it is a simple test involving scraping off cells from the cervix and examining them microscopically. The test is recommended to be carried out once a year to every three years – ask for your doctor's advice – to screen for early indications of this cancer; this is a form of preventive medicine. A good reason why it is important to have regular gyno check-ups, ladies.

It has long been known that this particular cancer is related to a woman's sexual behaviour, with early sexual intercourse and numerous sexual partners increasing her risk. It is now commonly detected in younger women and, worldwide, it is the second most common cancer in women. In 2006, a vaccine that is able to prevent infections from four strains of the sexually transmitted human papilloma virus came into use. This vaccine, administered over a period of six months, is for girls aged between 9 to 26. In 2007, a vaccine will be available for women up to the age of 55. It has been suggested that boys should also be vaccinated, as they are carriers of the virus; doing so would reduce the infection rate of HPV considerably.

BOWEL CANCER

Irritable bowel syndrome (IBS) and bowel cancer are on the rise, and diet and lifestyle play their part in these two diseases. Excessive consumption of processed foods, red meat and copious amount of alcohol eventually take their toll. According to the Institute of Cancer Research, up to 80% of colorectal cancers are diet related; if we included more fresh fruits, vegetable and fibre in our diet, we could start to feel better from the inside out! Bowel cancer can also be a 'family disease'; if close relatives develop bowel cancer before the age of 45 or if two or more family members have been diagnosed with bowel cancer, you will need to be more vigilant about what is going on inside your body. Pay a visit to the doctor's for advice on diet and lifestyle changes, as well as a rectal exam. There may not be any symptoms in the early stages, but take note of the following:

- Blood in the stools or mucus or black stools

- Changes in your normal bowel movements

- Long-term constipation or diarrhoea

- Pain and discomfort in the abdomen and back passage; persistent flatulence

- If there is a growth or obstruction in the bowel, you may feel sick and be constipated and bloated.

Make and keep an appointment with your doctor; it may not be cancer, but if a problem is detected early then there is a better chance of a positive outcome.

DIABETES

Type 2 diabetes is becoming increasingly common and can be seen in adults aged 35 and over, occasionally younger. Type 2 diabetes develops slowly and is due to the body not producing enough insulin. Below are some of the symptoms you should be aware of:

- increased thirst

- feeling tired; no energy

- weight loss

- frequent trips to the toilet, especially at night

- blurred vision

- infections such as thrush; urine and skin infections.

Weight is also a factor; if your waist measurement is over 31.5 inches for women (the toxic apple shape rears its head again), or 37.5 for a man, you could be at risk, especially if you:

- have a family history of diabetes

- have had diabetes during pregnancy (not men, of course!)

- are of Asian, African or Caribbean descent

- are not physically active.

Diabetes is diagnosed by measuring blood sugar levels. The two main tests that are used for diagnosing diabetes are performed separately, as one involves an overnight fast, after which the glucose levels in the blood are measured; if you have an elevated blood sugar level (above 140 mg/dl) on at least two occasions, it usually means you have diabetes. A normal reading is between 70–110 mg/dl.

The second test is the measurement of the body's ability to handle excess sugar after drinking a high-glucose drink. For this test, you need to have fasted for at least ten but not longer than sixteen hours. After an initial blood sugar reading, you are given a glucola bottle; this drink contains a high amount of glucose. Your blood will be tested thirty minutes after taking the drink and then after a one-, two- and three-hour period. During this time, you will need to be relaxed, either sitting or lying down.

The results are as follows: in a person who does not have

diabetes, the glucose levels in the blood rise following the glucose drink, but then fall quickly back to normal because insulin is produced in response to the glucose, and the insulin lowers the blood glucose. Someone who is presenting with diabetes has a higher glucose level, and the rate at which their levels fall is much slower, as either insulin is not being produced or, although it is being produced, the cells in the body do not respond.

Blood glucose measurements during the oral glucose tolerance test can vary, and the doctor may require you to take the test again. For both tests, your general health – illness can interfere with your blood sugar levels, as can certain medications such as steroids and diuretics – is taken into consideration and you need to be healthy and as active as you are in your normal daily routine to gain an accurate result.

Depending on the severity of the diabetes, it may initially be treated by altering your diet and getting more exercise, and your doctor or clinic will advise you, though there is plenty of information available. You may also need to take medication, usually in tablet form. Type 2 diabetes is a progressive disease and you may, at some point in the future, need insulin injections. Diabetes, over time, can cause other health problems, including heart disease, kidney failure, blindness, nerve damage, limb amputations and death. So it is important to manage your diabetes properly by following a healthy diet with regular check-ups; if you have any concerns about your health, get it checked out!

HEART DISEASE

As we pointed out in the 'Change-a-Pause' chapter, women are more protected during their fertile years than post-menopause, and many women assume breast cancer is their biggest risk factor when, in fact, they should be looking at heart disease.

Risk factors include:

- being overweight
- high or low cholesterol
- diabetes
- high blood pressure
- family history
- post-menopause
- smoking
- inactivity.

What can you do about any of the above? Conditions such as diabetes, hypertension and cholesterol can be present without you realising, though, once detected, they can be treated. Another good reason to do your yearly 'Well Woman' check!

Diet, exercise and smoking are all within your power to change, and, time and again, a balanced diet, including fresh fruits and vegetables, complex carbohydrates and foods high in Omega 3, oils such as salmon and sardines, keeps cropping up; doesn't that tell you something? Eating well and exercising equals better health. Any change to your diet and lifestyle is better than none at all.

If you have close relatives, parents or siblings who have heart conditions, inform your doctor and get the relevant checks done early; any conditions you have or are likely to develop can be monitored and treated, and, coupled with a good diet and exercise regime, you stand a better chance of managing any problems that may arise. There is little you can do about the menopause other than have the yearly Well Woman exam and be aware that your risk of heart disease has increased now that you are post-menopause. The main indication of heart disease is chest pain and shortness of breath; also, pain can be felt in the neck and jaw, upper back and abdomen, and you may experience tiredness, nausea, indigestion and sweating or feeling clammy. Though you may not have any of these symptoms and these symptoms may not mean heart disease, if you are feeling uncomfortable, don't dismiss it as 'nothing'; seek medical assistance. It may be nothing, but the sooner you receive treatment, the better. *Women die from heart disease.*

You must be holding your head in your hands, thinking that ageing has no benefits. Not so; a lot of the above can be contracted at any stage in life, and what you need to remember is that, almost on a daily basis, there are breakthroughs in preventative measures and treatment; it is possible that a lot of the above will not be considered so serious in the future. In the meantime take care of yourself, be informed and do not put off seeking treatment because you think the pains and twinges that you are having are nothing.

After reading the above, you probably think we should have entitled the book *Doom and Gloom*. But knowing about your own body and the possibility of developing any of the above not only empowers you to make lifestyle changes but gives you knowledge you can understand and work with. It is said that a little knowledge is a bad thing but no knowledge at all is worse! Oh, and don't forget diet and exercise (again). That's it – we've finished...

Stepping into the Future

With the onset of menopause, we know we are considered to be middle-aged; that, like it or not, is a fact. What is old age? Once upon a time, old age equated retirement, which was 60 for a woman (in the UK). Does that still apply today? For some, we are sure, it does, especially if you are not financially 'sound', as, according to the ELSA, the English Longitudinal Study on Ageing, England's poor and lonely face a higher death rate than wealthier people of the same age; wealth seems to equal a longer, healthier life. Accordingly, old age can be pushed back; some say 63 and others say it's 66. Maybe age does define us on the outside but a healthy mental attitude helps to keep us the age we feel. This line, in the future, will be even more clouded, as more over-60s will still be working and the lifestyle changes that are associated with turning from middle-aged to old-aged will not be so marked. There will be a continuation of activities, and, as long as we remain healthy in body and mind, there is no reason for that to change. Old age may then be defined by illness and incapacity, rather than a number.

Ageism

'Ageism' was not a word we had often come across, and we were surprised by the number of Internet sites that came up when we went in search of 'ageism' and its definition.

> AGEISM: attitudes and behaviours that belittle or discriminate against a person on the grounds of age. The term is used almost exclusively for younger people's treatment of older people.[7]

---

[7] Encarta, World English Dictionary, North American Edition, 2007.

Men and women over a certain age are seen as redundant; didn't we think the same when we were younger? Now, as we age, we do not want to be seen as having nothing to offer. Our accumulated knowledge can so often be portrayed negatively. Ageism is a recognised form of prejudice and as a consequence the respected 'elder' statesman/woman has lost his/her worth.

So, if you are over 50, are you more likely to be made redundant, refused a job because of your age or held back on the promotion ladder? Is the tide turning? We have heard a lot of people say they would rather employ an older workforce, as they tend to be more reliable, work-orientated and know how to make conversation with a customer, plus older women do not need maternity leave. Is that comment sexist or what?

From October 2006 in the UK, compulsory retirement below the age of 65 became unlawful and any retirements below that age now need to be justified. Check out www.agepositive.gov.uk; on redundancy, they state, 'Beware of losing the skills that your business needs. If you target older workers when selecting for redundancy, you may discover later that vital skills and company knowledge are lost.' This looks good for the future with regard to an older workforce. Maybe they should enforce an age limit for prime ministers and presidents: only those with relevant life skills, over the age of 55 and with immaculate credentials! Now there's food for thought.

The reality, of course, is that retirement, for so many people, is not an option, as they were born into poverty and will die in poverty, having spent a lifetime living hand to mouth from birth until death. What about the more wealthy societies? It is certainly no bed of roses, as an ever-growing number will still have mortgages or loans that need to be paid and many more just can't afford the luxury of retirement due to low or no available income. The option to continue working is double edged; many will have started their working life between the ages of 14 and 16 and the thought of working above the age of retirement because of financial necessity, either through their own mismanagement of funds or a pension that, nowadays, has less value than was hoped for, will, no doubt, leave some feeling bitter.

What about those of you who do not want to retire? Are you hoping to be given the opportunity to work until you choose otherwise? If you are self-employed, then the choice is yours, or are you now in a position of making choices that reflect what you want to do and not what you should do? What if you do have that choice? How would you address this choice? Do you continue working for as long as you are able, or could you use that time to volunteer your services and use your accumulated knowledge, built up over a lifetime, for the benefit of others? The only time you are eligible for a 'Life Diploma' is when you have lived a lifetime, and that cannot be bought – it is earned. The assets and knowledge we have are valuable; do not undermine or undersell yourself.

Growing Old (dis)Gracefully

As we grow older, we think we will have earned the right to be who we want and behave as we want, but we will be judged, and it will be the 'younger' generation – even our own children and grandchildren – who will judge us. (Can't you remember being a teenager and thinking anyone over 25 was past it?) If they are expecting 'Granny' to wear crimplene frocks and have a blue tint to her permed hair, like 'Gran' in the family photo album, then they are in for a shock. We will be reluctant to give up wearing the denims and trainers, and we will still be trying to fathom out our role in this ever-changing world.

Regardless, we think that our senior years (does that mean we have grown up?) will be a lot different to those of our parents and definitely our grandparents. Some of us are the swingers of the sixties – remember the sex, drugs and 'all we need is love' flower power? – while the rest of us are classed as the 'baby boomers', making us the skinheads and punks of the seventies, when parents despaired, wondering what kind of adults we would be. Well, we turned out to be the shakers and makers of today's society; mmm, maybe they were right! We were the lucky ones compared with today's kids; the majority of us will have grown up in a home with both parents present, and, though rebellious, we were taught our manners and did respect our elders. There was food on the table and we had the choice of either staying on at school and furthering our education or finding a job and becoming a trained and skilled member of the workforce.

Our senior years will not be ones spent in a rocking chair, slippers and cocoa by the fire – more likely a 'joint' and a bottle of red while relaxing on the decking! We may have taken up salsa dancing and kickboxing, but we would like to bet we will still be belting out Slade's 'Merry Christmas' on a yearly basis!

What celebrity role models do we have? Well, there is Paul McCartney and, of course, the Rolling Stones – or 'Strolling Bones', as the press refers to them. They were the 'hell raisers' of the sixties, and now they are all in their sixties, though they still play to packed audiences, the same group of fans that have been enjoying their music since their rise to fame. These die-hard fans stand shoulder to shoulder with a younger generation; music spans the age gap. What does that say about today's music and musicians? Will they still be performing in their sixties?

Joan Collins, Cher, Twiggy, Susan Sarandon… like them or not, they do not hide their age and are still making the most of their careers, and let's not forget Madonna: she reinvents herself, she entertains, writes, is an older mum, yet the media love to hate her. Why? Is it because she is rich and successful or because she is married to a younger guy? Or is it because she is not acting her age? Makes you think. And, while the press are decrying them, they are still raking in the money, so who has the last laugh?

We don't need to look at the celebrities who are out there, shaking a leg; what about closer to home? Older relatives and friends who enjoy life to the full and do not see themselves as old, only as old as they feel, 'only as old as the woman he is feeling' as the joke goes. They are the ones who know how to make the most of their life and are still having a good time, making friends, trying something new: they will probably tell you that this is the time of their life and any aches and pains are put to one side. These are now our role models, so take note. Will we follow their lead?

★ SMILE TIME ★

Looking Backwards

If you lived as a child in the forties, fifties, sixties or seventies, looking back, it's hard to believe that we have lived as long as we have…

As children, we would ride in cars with no seat belts or airbags. Our cots were covered with bright-coloured lead-based paint. We had no childproof lids on medicine bottles, doors or cupboards, and when we rode our bikes we had no helmets.

We drank water from the garden hose and not from a bottle. Horrors!

We would spend hours building go-carts out of scraps and then ride down the hill, only to find out we forgot the brakes. After running into the bushes a few times we learned to solve the problem.

We would leave home in the morning and play all day, as long as we were back when the street lights came on. No one was able to reach us all day.

No mobile phones. Unthinkable. We got cut and broke bones and broke teeth, and there were no lawsuits from these accidents. They were accidents. No one was to blame but us. Remember accidents?

We had fights and punched each other and got black and

blue and learned to get over it.

We ate sugary sweets, bread and butter, and drank cordial, but we were never overweight… we were always outside, playing. We shared one drink with four friends, from one bottle, and no one died from this.

We did not have Playstations, Nintendo 64, X-Boxes, video games, 250 satellite channels on TV, DVD movies, surround sound, personal mobile phones, personal computers, Internet chat rooms… we had friends. We went outside and found them. We rode bikes or walked to a friend's home and knocked on the door, or rung the bell, or just walked in and talked to them.

Imagine such a thing. Without asking a parent! By ourselves! Out there in the cold cruel world! Without a guardian – how did we do it?

We made up games with sticks and tennis balls, and ate worms, and although we were told it would happen, we did not put out very many eyes, nor did the worms live inside us for ever.

Footie and netball had tryouts and not everyone made the team. Those who didn't had to learn to deal with dis-appointment…

Some students weren't as smart as others and failed exams, so they were held back a year. Tests were not adjusted for any reason.

Our actions were our own. Consequences were expected. No one to hide behind.

The idea of a parent bailing us out if we broke a law was unheard of. They actually sided with the law – imagine that!

This generation has produced some of the best risk-takers and problem solvers and inventors, ever. The past fifty years have been an explosion of innovation and new ideas. We had freedom, failure, success and responsibility, and we learned how to deal with it all.

Anonymous

He's Under My Feet!

If you and your partner are newly retired, how do you accustom yourselves to this new-found freedom? For all of you out there who have hobbies and other regular social commitments, not having to work will give you more time to pursue the things that you enjoy.

The flip side to that coin may be that this is the first time in your lives you will be a couple together, at home, on a permanent basis, and it may be a shock to the system for you both. If you have always worked or had children, you will have been busy with all of the commitments that are part of raising a family and the chances are you have had little or no time together since you first became a courting couple. Don't count the holidays you have shared or the festive seasons, as these will have, no doubt, included other family and friends, and you can't necessarily count two weeks alone together as an indication of what your retirement will be like. And now that you have the rest of your lives looming in front of you, it's starting to look like the TV programme *One Foot in the Grave*, or, even worse, you find you have turned into Hyacinth Bucket!

It is not at all surprising that a lot of couples find this to be a turbulent time in their relationship and full of emotional strain. You could both be experiencing a loss of confidence in yourselves, as you now do not have a set role to follow. Let's face it, for most of our lives, there has been someone, if not telling us, then advising us what to do and when to do it, and now you are left to your own devices. Arguments about minute things that have never bothered you before (or was it because you did not notice them?) turn into long silences, and you feel as though you are vegetating and that life will consist of nothing more exciting than the weekly shop and watching the soaps on the TV.

Is this an exaggeration?

Not at all, as you now realise that this person you have lived with all of these years is someone you seem to have nothing in common with or you feel you no longer love. Can you get around this block? Communicating with each other is harder than it sounds; when did you last have a real heart-to-heart conversation, if at all? Now you may find you do not trust yourself to say the right words in the right way without each word sounding like a personal slur against their character. But, if you sit there without sharing your feelings, you will both become so despondent that you will be walking on eggshells and the 'our' time that you should be enjoying will feel like a prison sentence. In all probability, your partner will be feeling the same.

Someone has to make a move, and it could just be a case of finding some common ground and taking it from there. Maybe a trip down memory lane would be a good place to start – even the family photos. Photos bring back memories; it is surprising how we hold onto bitter memories but so easily forget the good times, and looking at the happy faces in your photographs does fill you with a warm glow, remembering all of those times spent with family and friends. This is what you should concentrate on: the good times in your relationship, because you can still have so many more. And, if you have been together for a number of years, you will surely have shared your hopes and dreams for the future, and now is the time to realise those dreams. If you still find it difficult to communicate, then get help: ask other family members or seek professional help. Don't wake up one day and realise you have wasted precious time on bickering and backbiting; life is far too short.

★ SMILE TIME ★

Two old pensioners are taking a trip down memory lane by going back to the place where they first met.

Sitting at a café, the little old man says, 'Remember the first time I met you, over fifty years ago? We left this café, went round the corner behind the gas works, and we made passionate love.'

'Why, yes, I remember it well, dear,' replies the little old lady with a grin.

'Well, for old times' sake, let's go there again and try again.'

The two pensioners pay their bill and leave the café. A young man sitting next to them has overheard their conversation and smiles to himself, thinking it would be quite amusing to follow the two old pensioners.

He gets up and follows them. Sure enough, he sees the two pensioners near the gas works. The little old lady gets herself ready and then reaches for the fence. Well, what follows is forty minutes of the most athletic action the man has ever seen. The little old folk set a pace that can only be described as phenomenal. Limbs are flying everywhere, the movement is a blur, and they do not stop for a single second. Finally, they collapse and don't move for an hour.

Well, the man is stunned. Never in his life has he ever seen anything that equates to this – not in the movies, not from his friends, not from his own experiences.

Reflecting on what he has just seen, he says to himself, 'If only I could carry on like that now, let alone in fifty years' time!'

The two old pensioners have, by this time, recovered and dressed themselves.

Plucking up courage, the man approaches the pensioners.

He says, 'Sir, in all my life I have never seen anybody act like that, particularly at your age. What's your secret? Was it like that fifty years ago?'

The pensioner replies, 'Son, fifty years ago, that fence wasn't electrified!'

Sadly, for some, retirement will bring illness and ruin all of those plans you had; the 'in sickness and in health' part of your marriage vows will be put to the test, and don't you just feel cheated? If there is anything to be learned by this, it is 'don't wait for your tomorrows if it is possible for you to carry out your plans today', at least you will have the memories to share together, rather than the 'if only'.

An important point to think about is your relationship with other people. Many couples are just that – a couple – and have no friends or outside interests other than each other, and that is great, but the point is, how will you cope alone? Regardless of your age or relationship with your other half, outside interests and friends can enrich your life, and this connection with the 'outside' will be priceless if you are left alone, because you will have people who not only share in your initial grief; they will be able to see you though the difficult step of being single, and friends or hobbies will still be there to support you when you feel ready to take that next step in your life.

Coping with bereavement is a hard road to travel, as it can leave you feeling alone, vulnerable and old; everything you look at or touch will bring the memories flooding back, along with the tears. It is natural and understandable to have a mourning period, and you may have a gamut of emotions and thoughts constantly running around inside your head, from despair to anger to feeling totally helpless; these emotions are normal. The months ahead, with all of those special events that you have shared, such as birthdays, anniversaries and Christmas, will feel especially difficult, as these tend to be family times and now part of the family will be missing. Depression can set in; for some, bereavement counselling will help, but the older you are, the harder it will be, and, until that time comes, not one of us knows how we will react. Often, you hear people talking about losing a loved one; some will say that they hope they are the first to 'go', as they don't know how they will cope, and yet others raise their eyes, trying to imagine their spouse being left alone and running a home. Death is a part of our life, and it is OK to think and talk about how you will face the future if you are left alone.

Miss Me, But Let Me Go

When I come to the end of the road,
And the sun has set for me,
I want no rites in a gloom-filled room;
Why cry for a soul set free?
Miss me a little, but not for long,
And not with your head bowed low.
Remember the love that once we shared.
Miss me, but let me go.
For this is a journey we all must take,
And each must go alone.
It's all part of the master plan,
A step on the road to home.
When you are lonely and sick at heart,
Go to the friends we know.
Laugh at all the things we used to do.
Miss me, but let me go.

Dating and Mating

There are a lot of people who have no problem living on their own, enjoying being able to do what they want, when they want to do it, especially if they have been at the beck and call of their spouse, as well as their children, for more years than they care to remember, and it will be a freedom that will not be given up lightly.

It was interesting to read through the 'lonely hearts' column in a magazine, the average age being 60. Men were looking for that 'special someone' with the possibility of an LTR (long-term relationship), while the women were looking for fun!

But there are many more who need the comfort and the familiarity of being a couple, and why not? Being alone and lonely can be a miserable existence.

So, where do you start? Well, there are plenty of groups that are aimed at singles – it's not just for the 18 to 30s. There are holidays, clubs and organised social events; it is out there if you can take that first step.

★ SMILE TIME ★

A very elderly gentleman (mid-90s), very well-dressed, hair well groomed, great-looking suit, flower in his lapel, smelling slightly of a good aftershave, presenting a well-looked-after image, walks into an upscale cocktail lounge.
Seated at the bar is an elderly-looking lady (mid-80s). The gentleman walks over, sits alongside her, orders a drink, takes a sip, turns to her and says:
'So, tell me, do I come here often?'

Will being older make you wiser when it comes to romance? Not necessarily, because you may just be looking for companionship, someone to go out with on social occasions, a friend, and, yes, some do feel the same way, but, as we said earlier, we are the children of the fifties, sixties and seventies and sex will still be high on the agenda, with a little help from Viagra!

If you think that you do not have anyone to please but yourself, think again, especially if you have children. Regardless of the fact that they are grown up with families and a social life of their own, they will vet your new beau and they will be worse than your parents. They will want to know all of the details and will be hoping he isn't after you for your money (don't forget your teenage years; he would have been after you for your body!). For all the women out there who are told, 'Hey, Mum, go for it,' there will be just as many told they are too old and not to make a fool of themselves; well, some kids still can't get their heads around their parents having sex, let alone enjoying it.

And don't presume he isn't married or involved with a significant other just because he is on the singles' scene. Some things don't change, and hearts can be broken at all ages.

Another important point to remember is not to be pushed into doing something you do not want to do; if you have said no to being intimate and he does not respect that, then send him on his way. And if he is insistent and again you have said no, remember: rape is rape and he is definitely not worth your time.

★ Smile Time ★

A couple, both aged 78, go to a therapist's office. The doctor asks, 'What can I do for you?'
The man says, 'Will you watch us have intercourse?'
The doctor looks puzzled, but agrees. When the couple finish, the doctor says, 'There's nothing wrong with the way you have intercourse,' and charges them £50.
This happened several weeks in a row. The couple would make an appointment, have intercourse with no problems, pay the doctor, and then leave.
Finally, the doctor asks, 'Just exactly what are you trying to find out?'
The old man replies, 'We're not really trying to find out anything. She's married and we can't go to her house. I'm married and we can't go to my house. The Holiday Inn charges £90. The Hilton charges £80. We do it here for £50, and I get £43 back from BUPA.'

What if you do find that certain someone for a romantic interlude? Is sex like riding a bike, where it all comes back to you as soon as you are in the saddle? You know the saying, there are plenty of good tunes played on an old fiddle. What if you are feeling body-conscious. If the only other person who has seen you naked is no longer around, how does it feel to bare all in front of someone new? Be confident in yourself; if you have reached this stage in your relationship, then it is by mutual consent. You don't necessarily have to be naked the first time you make love; treat yourself to some flattering lingerie and, if all goes well, baring all will be a natural progression of shared intimacy. Don't forget, most of us can make it look good with the right bra and M&S magic knickers, but remove them and it all heads south. Well, as long as he isn't some young buck with the body of a god, what are you worrying about? He will probably be as apprehensive as you when it comes to stripping off.

So there you are, ready, willing and able. Oh, you think, no worrying about an unwanted pregnancy – past all that now. Well, girl, you had better just stop yourself there and keep your knickers on. STDs (sexually-transmitted diseases) among the over-50s are becoming more commonplace and rising. Think chlamydia, syphilis, gonorrhoea, herpes; these can usually be cured, but HIV and AIDS have no known cure. Either be tactful and mention this or insist on condoms and no oral orientation. Age does not matter, and, if you are not 100% sure of your partner, practise safe sex.

Seriously, do consider your sexual health when embarking on a new relationship and, if you are worried, see your doctor.

According to AVERT:

> Few people would picture the face of HIV as a wrinkled one. Yet older people across the world face many unique challenges as a result of the spread of HIV: in prevention, in diagnosis, in the necessity of caring for others and in the loss of those around them.

It goes on to say:

> In the USA, 10–15% of all reported new HIV infections occur among people over the age of 50, with a quarter of these among the over-60s. This amounted to around 78,000 people in April 2005, and the percentage of new infections occurring in this age group are rising. This is an increase of 18,000 people or 30%. In the UK, current data suggest that 8% of adults living with HIV or AIDS fall into the over-50 age category.

We haven't finished yet; carry on reading…

> Studies show that infection rates are not concentrated around the lower end of the age group but spread across people in their 50s, 60s and 70s fairly evenly. Despite the stereotype of older people as abstinent, many are sexually active and some are injecting drug users. As women pass childbearing age they are less likely to use a condom during sex, as it is not required for contraceptive purposes. After the menopause a natural thinning of the vaginal walls occurs in many women and lubrication reduces, causing an increased risk of tearing during intercourse and making older women more susceptible to HIV infection.

There's more…

> The assumption that older people are not sexually active often prevents an early diagnosis of HIV. Older people may be reluctant to talk to doctors about their sex lives and medical professionals may be reluctant to ask the right questions. This often results in the overlooking of possibilities that an older person might have come into contact with HIV, and HIV testing will not be thought necessary. The lack of understanding of the virus amongst older people, in high-income countries, such as the UK, and in low-income countries,

makes them less likely to come forward for testing, as they do not believe that they could be at risk of contracting the virus.

Often the idea that an older patient might have contracted HIV will be the last possibility investigated when all other options have been exhausted. The symptoms that an older person with HIV presents with, such as fatigue, weight loss, poor memory, skin rashes and swollen lymph nodes, can be seen in many other illnesses typically associated with ageing, resulting in frequent misdiagnosis.[8]

What is Safe Sex?

Practising safe sex may sound boring, but it could save your life and, if you consider yourself to be health-conscious and informed on feminine health matters, you need to make sure safe sex with casual partners is a priority.

- Safe sex isn't just for the teenagers.

- Use a condom and a lubricating gel. If you suffer vaginal dryness gel will guard against tears to the vagina and anus.

- Use a fresh condom if you have vaginal sex following anal sex, as anything lurking in the anus can be passed into the vagina.

- A condom should be worn during oral sex.

- Cleaning teeth and using a mouthwash before oral sex will cut down the possibility of passing on any infections.

- Cover sores or cuts on fingers.

- Sex aids should always be thoroughly washed and not shared.

- Safe sex applies to same-sex as well as heterosexual contact.

---

[8] www.avert.org; AVERT is an international HIV and AIDS charity based in the UK, with the aim of averting HIV and AIDS worldwide.

Just remember: if you can't be good, be careful, as our mothers used to say.

★ SMILE TIME ★

Mary and Sheila are outside their old people's nursing home
having a smoke, when it starts to rain. Sheila pulls out a condom,
cuts off the end, puts it over her cigarette and continues smoking.
Mary: What's that?
Sheila: A condom. This way, my cigarette doesn't get wet.
Mary: Where did you get it?
Sheila: You can get them at any chemist.
The next day, Mary hobbles into the local chemist and
announces to the pharmacist that she wants a box of condoms.
The guy, obviously embarrassed, looks at her kind of strangely
(she is, after all, over 80 years of age) but very delicately asks
what brand she prefers.
Mary: Doesn't matter, son, as long as it fits a Camel.

And you thought getting older would be boring; if anything, it sounds more complicated, but, hey, enjoy the journey and enjoy your life.

Addressing the Future

On the questionnaire that we sent out and when talking with women about their future, the fear that surfaced was that of old age and the associated problems: illness, loss of partner, lack of funds, dementia and the thought of ending life in a nursing home as a forgotten 'vegetable'. Well, except for one woman who feared her mother-in-law was going to outlive her… The concerns are justified, especially in a society where 'youth culture' rules. When you are fit and healthy, you are by no means over the hill, regardless of your age, and, generally, we are healthier than previous generations, as we have access to better medical care, and we are living longer than our predecessors. But is the media responsible in leading us to believe that we have nothing to look forward to as we age? The doom-and-gloom headlines, such as 'pensioner mugged', 'eighty-year-old raped and murdered' or 'neglect of our old in hospitals' and 'near starvation in nursing homes', are enough to make us all cringe at the prospect of ageing. Yes, we need to be made aware of these things and the abuse is dreadful, but does reading these headlines make us fearful of our future?

Let's address some of those fears that are lurking in the darkest corners of our minds. It is generally acknowledged that, in a couple who are of a similar age, it will be the male who dies first. Realistically, this is one thing you have no control over and 'control' is the key word as to how we see our future. We have had control over our own lives for so long that the thought of not being able to make our own decisions about our life is fearful. Do not let this fear mar your outlook; you may not be able to see into the future, but there are a lot of things you can do now to safeguard it. It is not a case of being morbid; it is a practical approach to getting the future you want if, at some point, you do become incapable of making decisions.

It is essential to make a will. If you own property or have other assets and monies in the bank, making a will gives you the say as to how your assets are to be shared. How will the local dog's home know they were supposed to be the main beneficiary if you did not make it clear? Consult a legal professional and get some peace of mind; these things are not set in stone and can be altered if your circumstances change or you are not happy with your original decisions. UK assets held jointly, such as houses and bank accounts, will automatically pass to the surviving spouse, but anything held in one name only, if a will has not been made, will be distributed in accordance with intestacy rules and may go to other family members – so make a will!

Due to all of the developments in health care, more lives

are being saved, and the same technology can be used to keep a person alive even though there is no chance of recovery. If you have strong feelings about your medical care should you become hospitalised or terminally ill, if possible, make a living will. A living will gives you the say on the medical treatment you wish or do not wish to receive. These are legally binding documents in the UK (and, we assume, many other countries as well) and are recognised by the British Medical Association, the Royal College of Nursing, the General Medical Council, the Nursing and Midwifery Council, the Law Society, and Age Concern.

Take time out to address these matters with your family, because, if no such form is in place, your family will not have any legal right to act on your behalf with regard to treatment being given or withheld. It is understandable that this is quite a difficult decision to make and not to be taken lightly, but it will save your family a lot of heartache in these situations if they know they are following your wishes. Living wills state your refusal or acceptance of treatment and cannot be used to actively end a life.

You may see this as a form of suicide. It isn't. If it wasn't for modern technology, you would not have to think about this issue. This is not a problem that many of our parents or grandparents faced; if you went into a coma or suffered heart failure or stopped breathing, you died, usually sooner rather than later, and it was accepted that this was 'what they would have wanted', so what's changed? Nothing, really, except that oxygen can be pumped into your body, giving the appearance of life, and only you can decide what you consider to be 'quality of life'.

You may or may not have close family members to aid you in making decisions. That isn't a problem. There are options available to you. You can appoint a designated person or persons to act on your behalf; they can be family, friends or legal professionals, they can have your Power of Attorney as follows:

1. Power of Attorney is a legal document that allows someone to act on your behalf in making decisions and signing legal documents if you are not able, either through illness or living abroad, and would be treated as such in a court of law.

2. An Enduring Power of Attorney is a legal document that enables you to have 'attorneys' acting on your behalf to manage any property and finances, not health and well-being. Again, this is a legal document, but it does not have to be registered with the OPG – Office of the Public Guardian – unless stipulated by you. Otherwise, it will only be registered if you lose the capacity to make decisions or no longer wish to deal with your own affairs.

3. You will, however, from 2007, if the law is passed, be able to make a Lasting Power of Attorney; again, this is a legal document allowing attorneys to act on your behalf – possibly two documents: one for finance and property and a separate one for personal health and welfare. The attorneys can be family, friends or professionals and be one or more people. A Lasting Power of Attorney cannot be used until it has been registered with the OPG, where it will be given a legal seal. Even when the document has been registered, as long as you are able, your attorneys should involve you in any decision making. You also have the right to stop a Lasting Power of Attorney as long as you are able to make that decision, and your attorneys also have the right to change their mind; this will not affect the document if you have more than one attorney in place. As a safeguard, you will need to inform up to five people before the document is registered and they will have the right to object – they may feel you have been pressured into this decision or the document is not in your best interests.

Though it sounds complicated, it is better to be reassured that any decisions you have made are the right ones for you and that you are not being exploited. Consult a legal professional, contact the Department of Constitutional Affairs or check out relevant web sites.

Now that you are feeling suitably depressed, let's carry on. At some point in your future, you may require 24-hour care. Again, discuss what you would want with your family, friends, attorneys. If it is your wish to remain in your own home, nursing agencies can provide the care you need; it will be expensive, but home nursing gives you the opportunity to remain in familiar surroundings. You may be entitled to care through the social services; if you contact the Commission for Social Care, they can provide advice and details about care services.

You may choose to go into a nursing home; let's face it, for the ones that get bad press, there are good care homes out there, where you will be in a safe environment with the facilities you require. You may also have company, should you choose, and that is a consideration if you do not like the idea of being home alone. Again, private nursing homes can be costly, and, with residential social care, your financial circumstances are taken into consideration.

It may be that your family wishes to care for you. In many cultures, parents are still revered and respected and it would be unthinkable not to care for them as they age, but ours is a changing society and, as much as we love our kids and they love us, this may not be practical. There is a lot to be considered with this arrangement; any niggles and fallouts you may have had over the years are still going to be there, and, no matter how well things start off, they can soon spiral downwards due to misunderstandings or disagreements on the home front. If there is a possibility of having your own space within the household or an annex being built so there is a division of 'home', this makes sense, as all parties can keep a certain amount of independence and privacy while having the knowledge that there is someone close by. A household of noisy teenagers, TVs and music blaring is not a formula for success when all you want is a little peace and quiet.

Abuse of the elderly is rising; elder abuse is defined as 'a single repeated act or lack of appropriate action, occurring within any relationship where there is an expectation of trust, which may cause harm or distress to an elder person.'[9]

Get the information you need, as help and assistance, both financial and practical, are available, and this could make all the difference in making an arrangement like this work. It is acknowledged that home carers are unsung heroes, *but* living within a family unit that is built on love, trust and respect – well, no amount of money can buy that kind of care and peace of mind.

No, no, don't put the book down; we may as well finish what we have started, and in this case, we need to address the final resting place. Do you know what you want to be done with your bodily remains? Do you carry an organ donor card? If you do, then you have considered and made decisions about your death and helping others. What about funeral arrangements? Do you want one that will reflect your religious beliefs and want to be buried accordingly? Or would you rather be cremated? Would you like to leave your body to medical science or be frozen in a cryonic pod, awaiting the future? Are you a conservationist who wishes to be buried in a biodegradable coffin and commemorated by having a tree planted above you? Or would you like your ashes scattered on your favourite football team's pitch? Do something; don't be indifferent. Let your nearest and dearest know of your wishes and it will take the burden from their shoulders. We are so 'anti'-death in this day and age, yet, in life, it is our only certainty. It can be liberating to face your future and your demise, because once you have, you can get on with living.

---

[9] www.elderabuse.org.uk.

Home Base

What about your home? Are you happy there? If you want to carry on living in your own home, take a look at what can be done to make life easier in the future, should the need arise. Is the house you are in too big for your needs? Can you down-size, keeping your independence? What can you do to make your home user-friendly? There are a lot of aids, such as stair lifts – how cool will your grandkids think you are? You can find walk-in showers, as well as other specially adapted home appliances. More items are now becoming available as the manufacturers are coming to understand the growing number of older people, the ageing 'baby boomers' and their spending power. To quote: 'You can sell a young man's car to an old man, but you can't sell an old man's car to anybody.' It is all to do with our concept of age and how old we see ourselves; we may need these items to enable us to be more independent, but we don't necessarily want them to be labelled as such, and designers realise that we want style, not just functionality, so items are being sold as 'ergonomically' designed with comfort in mind. Well, if the cap fits…

Despite the many who will be able to receive aid from the social services, there are many more who do not fall into that category, usually because they have, on paper, healthy finances. Will you be prepared to spend that money on receiving care by employing someone to clean and prepare a meal for you, or even employing a live-in 'companion' to give day-to-day assistance? If money is a concern and you own your own property, consider taking advantage of equity release; this is now becoming a popular choice. If it means keeping your independence as well as having access to your money, do it. Forget about leaving an inheritance; you have earned this money, no doubt by going without just so you could have a nest egg – enjoy and make use of it.

As well as council-run facilities offering sheltered accommodation for older people, there are now more private houses being built with the over-55s in mind, giving you independence and security in a 'stylish community of similar-minded people'. These, of course, vary in price depending on the location and the amenities offered; some are also retirement homes with features such as serviced living, while others offer nursing care. This is a good option if you want to remain in the same place or you know that, in the future, you or your partner will need 24-hour nursing care. And, while some may love their neighbours, there are many more who don't want to live next door to a young family and noisy kids. Are we selfish? If we are, put it down to our age.

There is an ever-increasing number of people choosing to retire abroad; if that is your plan, then you need to 'read between the lines' before you pack your bags. The Foreign and Commonwealth Office gives all of the relevant information about retiring abroad, such as your right to live in any EEA area; these are countries that are full members of the European Union. There is information on your welfare rights abroad as well as medical care, but it does stress getting health insurance to cover medical costs, dental costs and medical repatriation. Another important point is making a will in the country you will be living in regarding any property and monies held there; your consul should be able to provide you with a list of reputable lawyers to help you in this matter. You will, no doubt, have some idea as to your income when you retire, and, if you are eligible for a state pension, which you will receive if you live abroad, you need to be aware that you may not receive annual increments if you are not covered by EC social security regulations. There is also information on tax liability and the benefits of offshore banking.

Don't forget the Internet. Not computer-savvy? That really isn't a problem; there are a lot of courses on offer and, if it means being independent, you will master the computer. It will give you the freedom to do your banking, pay bills and do the weekly shopping online; you can browse at your leisure and at a time that is convenient to you. Not only does the Internet offer you the chance to research your favourite hobby or trace your family tree, you can download newspapers and books or listen to music, and you can keep in contact with family and friends. There is no need to be lonely, especially if you have a web camera or a video link facility, and don't forget all those chat rooms; you would be surprised by how many people are out there, 'chatting'.

There are also many financial perks for the over-55s; you will get better deals on house and car insurance as well as travel, etc. Many companies know the spending power you have, and they want your cash, especially in a credit card debt-ridden society, so let your age and your cash avail you of a bargain.

The above is aimed at showing you that you can have control over your life as you become older. The majority of women who answered our questionnaire were looking forward to the future and to the chance to live the life they wanted but, if you thought this chapter was getting a bit too heavy, we thought we would go in search of a little light relief. We did not have to look far; one web site gave us enough information to make even the most sceptical of you take note: www.direct.gov.uk/Over50s.

This one site will take you from learning how to use the computer, at no cost to you, to finding courses at colleges and universities, if you fancy a change in direction or just for the sake of learning something new. With some of the courses, you do attend college or university; others are distance learning courses. Some of these are free; others can be paid a term at a time, or, if you are on a low income, you may be eligible for financial assistance.

You can find out about job training or retraining in your area, how to put a CV together, applying for jobs and interview techniques. There is even advice on setting up your own business. See? We keep telling you: you are never too old.

You can take a look at your pension forecast as well as looking at ways to enhance your income in retirement, or, if you are on a low income, what benefits you may be entitled to receive.

It won't be a case of what to do with your spare time; it will be a case of not having enough time to pursue all that is on offer when you are armed with the information on leisure pursuits.

They also take a look at both women's and men's health, in the health and well-being section, as well as giving contact details for more organisations than we knew existed. If you fancy volunteering, there are numerous areas where you can use your skills, locally or even abroad, though sometimes just being available to chat or even to pour someone a cup of tea is of more help than we realise.

If you think your life does not matter and that's how you see your future, then it will be a long and probably boring retirement. Health-wise, the more active you are physically and mentally, the better quality of life you will have, but that applies to every one of us, regardless of age. Attitude defines us more than age, and, if you are able to step into the future in a positive and confident manner, the world is your oyster.

Finally, a quote by Rebeck on ageing: 'Women get facelifts. And men get cute little girlfriends.' What he didn't know was that, along with the facelift, a stint down at the gym and breast implants, we can also have a 'toy boy'.

These are sites worth looking at. Don't pull a face because you think you are not *that* age; these sites are full of information on more topics than you can imagine:

- www.citzensadvice.org.uk
- www.helptheaged.org.uk
- www.heyday.org.uk
- www.agepositive.gov.uk
- www.saga.co.uk
- www.careaware.co.uk

Media and All That Jazz

We will be honest and admit we are influenced by the media: a lot of our discussions are based on what we have read, seen or heard; then we will agree, disagree or debate the relevance of the so-called 'facts'. And, at the risk of sounding shallow, we do take note of cosmetic ads, especially when it comes to skin-care products – well aren't we all looking for that miracle face cream?

If you say you are not influenced by advertisements, think again. In this ever-changing society, perfection is craved, a certain lifestyle is portrayed and you may be unaware of the information that you are taking in. We are being told what to think, feel, eat and wear, what size we should be, and, if we don't fit their criteria, it can leave some of us feeling fearful, stupid, ugly and fat. The sad part is that the one who is unhappy about themselves or their lifestyle is the intended 'victim'. And you can be a victim in more ways than one. Selling a perfect lifestyle also leads to debt: spend today, worry tomorrow – why shouldn't you have it all?

To achieve the looks and the lifestyle costs money, but that isn't a problem, credit cards are available at every shop. Loans for cars, furniture and holidays leave you owing more than you are earning, and the only ones to suffer are you and your family. When did you last see an advertisement in a glossy magazine showing the debt collector calling and removing items from a home, or a house being repossessed and the family made homeless? What about someone taking their own life because they can no longer afford their 'lifestyle'? The suicide victim often takes their life not just because of mounting debt; how can they face family and friends who think they are successful, only to find it is really nothing but a façade? How tragic for all involved.

Advertisements are made with the sole purpose of selling that particular product and/or lifestyle. Look around you; how many billboards do you see that advertise healthy food and diet? Not many, but the billboards are flooded with advertisements for fast food. The interesting part is that, next to it, you will have a super-thin model looking suitably disinterested, displaying clothes few of us normal-sized women could wear or afford. Stop and think for a minute: what does this picture tell you? Eat junk food and stay thin? What a contradiction; we all know that junk food is not good for us, and you certainly will not stay thin, or healthy, for long if you indulge in too much junk food.

On the other hand, who said you have to be thin? Who has set these standards? We all know that being overweight is bad for our health, but do we know what a healthy weight is if we take into consideration height, bone density, age, muscle-to-fat ratio, etc.? Let's be honest: we women are our worst enemy, and we do put tremendous pressure on ourselves regarding how we should look; these thoughts have been shaped by what we see. Have you ever heard a man asking another man what size clothes he wears? We accept that we come in different heights and colours, so why can't we accept different shapes and size as well? Is it our need to conform to what we think society wants, or are we conforming to the media standard?

It has long been noted that the stick-thin fashion models are not positive role models for young girls; it is all but impossible to adapt your body shape to the ones you emulate. Believe it or not, in Hollywood, being a size 10 is a no-no; all want to be a size 0 – that's a UK size 4 – and Victoria Beckham's waspish, 23-inch waist is now craved by women as well as young girls.

What about older women? It is now common to find mature women standing in line with the young teens who are suffering with anorexia and bulimia, not to mention BDD (body dysmorphic disorder). Not heard of that one? Well, neither had we. It is considered a serious psychiatric illness, and Mind, the mental health charity, estimates that BDD affects 1% of the population and is most common in women and adolescents. BDD sufferers are not happy with the way they look; this may be weight, height, hair or any other body part, and the 'problem' can be real or imagined.

Interestingly, a large beauty product manufacturer completed a survey involving 3,300 girls and women, in ten countries, aged between 15 and 64. 90% were not happy with their body weight and 67% withdraw from day-to-day activities because of their looks.[10]

Women are being led to believe that 50 is the 'new' middle age, but the reality is that it is still 40. Why? Well, the words 'middle-aged' should give you a clue; we are in the middle of our lifespan. It is possible that we may live until we are 80-plus, so 40 is the onset of middle age. Our bodies tell us this, and that is why we start to physically change, winding down from our productive years; this is nature doing what it does best, and, although it can be tampered with, as yet it cannot be permanently changed.

We live in a society that glamorises youth and beauty, and, as we age in years, so does our body; some women are lucky and their beauty seems ageless, but the majority of us out there need a little help. When we look at images and articles of women, usually celebrities – and we are talking about the ones aged over 40 – what do we actually see? Well, if the article is 'selling' us a product or advertising an opening night, a book she has written (especially if it is of the lurid kind) or even a charity that this celebrity is involved with, we see a siren. Her age is a feature of the article because she looks so good; there are no visible wrinkles, make-up and hair are immaculate, and

---

[10] www.campaignforrealbeauty.co.uk.

the clothes and shoes – well, definitely more than a month's wage for most of us. And, to cap it all, she has a figure that is enviable. So we read or even scan the article/image, digesting some, dismissing other parts, and turn over the page, either vowing to get on the treadmill and 'work that body' or thinking, 'Well it's OK for them – isn't it!'

What does the above leave you thinking? Could it be, 'I'm that age, why don't *I* look so good?' or 'Why have I got spots and fluid retention? Why do I always wear clothes that have elastic waists?' Maybe not, but we bet you linger a few moments on that image, subconsciously thinking, 'If only…'

But look in those same newspapers and magazines, and you will see how they delight in showing images of the same 'star' caught at a time when she is just getting on with her everyday life. Her hair is a mess, she is not wearing make-up, and just look at her wrinkled neck and jowls! The clothes she is wearing look like they came from a jumble sale, and her figure is not as slender and toned as previously portrayed. How does that make you feel? We become a little outraged; any one of us can look like a star with the entire make-up and costume department working on achieving the right look, and, of course, the magic of the computer and airbrushing. This is the technique used to make the most of what we have or no longer possess: flawless skin, a wrinkle-free neck, sparkling eyes and curves that would guarantee us centre page in any man's magazine! Do we blame the 'stars'? No. They are doing what the majority of us do: they are earning a living, and, they like us, we are sure, would rather see an image of groomed perfection than the reality.

That is just one example of media at work. Our next also gives food for thought. There are, according to an article we read,[11] 72 million women aged between 40 and 59 in Europe, and the article goes on to say, 'Millions are using their 40s and 50s to rediscover themselves.' Excuse us? Millions?

---

[11] Judith Woods, 'Mid-life crisis? Bring it on!', *Healthy*, Issue 42, March 2006.

No doubt a large number of these women would like to 'rediscover' themselves in order to escape the life they live. We should consider ourselves lucky in that we can make decisions and have choices, but even that sometimes has to be 'configured' around personal life and family commitments. Financially, what most of us are able to do and what we would like to do are not always the same, and we juggle our available cash on a weekly or monthly basis. Yet we are led to believe that we have freedom of choice. Well, we do not know of anyone who is totally 'free'; even if we do not confine ourselves, the societies that we live in do and we are all bound by the law of the land.

Seriously, our thoughts do go out to all of those, not just women, who are stuck in a trap that may include poverty, abuse and a lack of knowledge or being confined in a society that does not respect human rights. That said, it does make sense that women who do have the chance to follow another life path are often aged 40 and upwards. They will have reached midlife and may have the opportunity, now that the family has grown up, to look at other careers or pursue a long-held dream. For others, a long-term relationship ends and they find they can enjoy a new-found independence where they can please themselves; in their doing so, their actions speak volumes. Of all those many, many others whose lives will still be the same, are they resentful of women who *do* have the opportunity for change, and, if so, is this resentment fuelled by what they read or see?

Let's go back a few years and take a look at the women born in the late 1940s and onwards who found they did not have to follow their pre-destined role as previously set out. We are talking about the role of wife, mother and homemaker. It was all so clear-cut at one time: if you married, you gave up your job and concentrated your efforts on home and family. When the children were grown up and married with their own families, you were a grandparent, a pensioner and then dead, which is a simplistic way of looking at it. So is our dissatisfaction due to the fact that we no longer have a set role? We burnt our bras and now we are paying the price? Or can we say our lives have been influenced by advertising and the media? For many, the dream of a better life that is promised if only you do this or become that is a dream that has never materialised, and, when the bubble finally bursts, who is to blame, if anyone, and who picks up the pieces?

We were not born when the first televisions, only available in black and white, started to make an appearance in households (early 1950s) and we did not know the world was our oyster until we saw the world on the TV and read about it in newspapers and lifestyle magazines. We are talking about the ones that showed you holidaying in Spain and – shock horror – discussed sex before marriage! (As if couples had never walked down the aisle anything less than virgins.) We became sexually liberated with the advent of the 'pill'; one-night stands were fine, and smoking a joint was considered the norm. It was OK to set up home with your boyfriend, and we were told how he was the 'new man' and would be sharing the household chores and cooking. Well, there's food for thought. Agree or disagree, it is a fact that a woman's role has changed but some of us still aren't quite sure what it is or should have been.

One thing that does not change, though I'm sure the scientists have tried: women are still the ones who grow and nurture a foetus and give birth, though, nowadays, we don't even need a man in our life, as IVF is the one-stop shop for all your baby needs: blue eyes, blond hair, a dimpled chin and an IQ to match!

We are ridiculed for opting for caesarean delivery rather than the push, shove and grunt type, and we are less than perfect if we do not breastfeed and bond with our offspring and – shame, shame, shame! – we are too eager to get back to work, leaving the fruit of our loins to be (mis)cared for in nurseries or by childminders. These are not our words.

Women are being put down on a daily basis, and, when we are looking for a bit of light relief in the daily paper or turn on the TV, we are told the blame is firmly on our shoulders when it comes to children being misfits of society, due to:

- not being part of a two-parent family

- mothers going out to work

- our lack of parenting skills.

There's no wonder women wore shoulder pads in the eighties; it wasn't power dressing – they were necessary to carry the guilt around. We did and do not consciously set out to do things wrong; it's just that no one gave us the correct manual – and, as it has turned out, there wasn't one then and there isn't one now; just lots of information that is right one week and wrong the next. All we ever really did or do is follow the trends as laid out before us in black and white.

Though we are still told the world is our oyster, it isn't available to us all, and many of those who have 'sampled a cookie' are looked down on because they choose not to conform to the stereotypical female role. It is no secret that girls are outperforming the boys in schools, and they are the ones taking up the once male-dominated professions of law, medicine and 'big business'. There are now more female millionaires than ever and the number is rising. Do they have to make sacrifices for earning that kind of money? The answer is yes. Compare successful businessmen with successful businesswomen. A man can still have it all: job, wife and family – yet, he does not have to juggle these three things, whereas the successful woman has to:

- find a partner who does not begrudge her her success and is not threatened by her wealth;

- find the time to become pregnant – providing her biological clock is still ticking – and hopefully not spend nine months throwing up or suffering any complications;

- take maternity leave without losing her status or business;
- run the home;
- still be a sex siren, mother, housewife and career girl;
- not feel guilty when she can't stay at home if her child has measles, mumps or a cold.

And you thought 'superwoman' went out with the nineties! She is still there; it's just that she has to keep her head down and get on with it. 'I have yet to hear a man ask for advice on how to combine marriage and a career' (Gloria Steinem).[12]

Respect is earned; we don't doubt that, but women who are good at what they do struggle to make it to the top of their career ladder, while, if they took off their blouse for a topless photo or were someone's mistress, they are guaranteed instant fame. Their image will be in every paper and, depending on who they've slept with, maybe on the news as well. What information does that send to the girls still growing up? In reality, nothing has changed in years; women still fight for the right to be accepted and boys still prefer blondes with big tits. Yet we profess to be confident within and comfortable with ourselves as we are; if that is so, why are Botox and silicone the 'gods' some of us worship? Read on…

Keeping 'Abreast' of Changes

Once upon a time, not so long ago, most of us did not know anyone who had had cosmetic surgery; over the last few years, that has changed, and, if we don't personally know them we know of women who have had breast implants, dermabrasion, tummy tucks or a face lift. A few years ago, if someone had said, 'Will you have plastic surgery in the future?' the answer

---

[12] Gloria Steinem has been involved for over thirty years as a feminist activist, organiser, writer and lecturer.

would have been, 'Don't be silly.' One of the questions on our questionnaire was, 'Would you consider cosmetic surgery?' The majority said, 'No.' That led us to thinking: what do we see as being cosmetic enhancement? We use the word 'enhancement' because it is not always necessary to go under the surgeon's knife to have a cosmetic procedure.

What are contact lenses if not cosmetic? How about a visit to the dentist: would you like them whitened, straightened, bridged or implanted? Not cosmetic? A visit to the hairdresser's: highlights, low lights, semi-permanent or permanent colour, hair extensions, permanent wave or the latest cut. Not cosmetic? Nail extensions, pedicure, manicure, false eyelashes. Not cosmetic enhancements? Of course they are; it is just that we are so used to these enhancements that we do not necessarily see them as anything other than part and parcel of our life; they help improve our appearance and give us a 'feel-good' factor.

As girls, we couldn't wait to get our first eyeshadow, usually blue, and mascara, and (we should have listened to Mum) to shave our legs. If anyone asked us now, 'Would you consider cosmetic enhancement?', the answer would be, 'Yes, why not?' Why? For exactly the same reasons we used our first eyeshadow and nail polish: the feel-good factor and the fact that, as adolescents, we could advertise, via our painted faces and pouting lips, that we were all grown up.

When we watch TV or pick up a magazine, what are we seeing? At one time, films, TV soaps, etc., were the product of art imitating life; don't you think this has now reversed and life imitates what we see and read? Our readiness to accept cosmetic surgery is again due to the media – where would Pamela Anderson and Katie Price, AKA 'Jordan', be without their 'enhancements'? Probably not on the front covers of the glossy magazines. Most of us love to have a look at the 'celebs' and their lives as featured in *Hello* and *OK*; it is a bit of escapism from everyday life and possibly the reason we now accept that we can have the 'Hollywood white smile' and breasts that do not deflate when lying down. Because we do take note of what and who is around us, we are led to believe that being a 'certain age' means you are no longer viable, and, God forbid, we should look our age. They say beauty is skin deep; well, with 'cosmetic enhancement' you can change that on a regular basis. You can be whatever age you want and have the look you want, choose the nose, lips, bum and boobs out of a catalogue on the doctor's desk, and why not? There are lots of reasons why not. As mentioned, older women who are anorexic or bulimic are in danger of taking their obsession with slimness to an early grave. Breast enhancement, if not done correctly, can leave you looking like Quasimodo, though the 'hump' is in the wrong place; worse, the implanted breasts could leak, causing serious medical problems, and that equates to more surgery, possible disfigurement or your life. Botox and collagen injections, if not administered properly/hygienically – don't forget, Botox is a poison – can leave you looking and no doubt feeling like a freak, and a facelift can leave a woman looking like a fish out of water, and none of the above is guaranteed to make you feel good on the inside, where it counts. Enhancements, if done for the right reasons or for a genuine cosmetic need, are beneficial, but they will not necessarily give your confidence a boost or make you socially acceptable.

The reality is that the cosmetics industries and plastic surgeons are seeing an increase in their sales, and women as well as men of any age are a target. Young girls want to look like their favourite model, singer or actress, and they know it can be achieved with a nip, snip and a tuck, while the older ones want to look younger. Are we frightened of growing old or looking our age? Who are we competing with: the younger generation or our mothers? Take away the hair colour and the modern blow-dried hairstyle, wipe off the make-up – whose face would we see in the mirror? Our mum's? Is that so bad?

It would be interesting to look upon the bathroom shelves and dressing tables and in the make-up bags of the women who say they are not influenced by the media and advertising. We don't think they will be using the same products they used as teenagers; you tend to buy products appropriate to your skin type and age, whether that is a conscious decision or not. Only they know, but, if they are not influenced by advertising, I hope the advertisement firms are taking note, as their clients must be wasting millions.

Do the above remarks mean we are anti-media? Of course not. Are advertisements and the media good for us? Well, we all like to be informed and to know what the market has to offer, and we all like to have choices. But our advice is: start to think and question things, make your own decisions. It is so easy to go with the flow and be 'brainwashed' by the glitz and glamour and promises of a lifestyle that, for many, only exists in their dreams.

Instead, why can't we be reasonable to each other and comment more on the goodness of heart and inner beauty – the souls? Real happiness and beauty does come from within; contentment and being at ease with yourself cannot be bought at any price.

These are the words of Audrey Hepburn, the actress, when asked to share her beauty tips.

> For attractive lips, speak words of kindness.
> For lovely eyes, seek out the good in people.
> For a slim figure, share your food with the hungry.
> For beautiful hair, let a child run his/her fingers through it once a day.
> For poise, walk with the knowledge that you never walk alone.
> People, even more than things, have to be restored, renewed, revived, reclaimed, and redeemed; never throw out anyone.
> Remember, if you ever need a helping hand, you will find one at the end of each of your arms.
> As you grow older, you will discover that you have two hands; one for helping yourself, and the other for helping others.

Even so, we like to look good, and most of us would like to get rid of those telltale lines and age signs. So, if you fancy toning up a few of those wrinkles but cannot afford the cream or the Botox injections or will not spend your cash on principle, here are a few tips, 'au naturel' of course (as seen in the beauty column of the local paper – told you we were shallow). [13]

- Tip your head back, looking at the ceiling; place your bottom lip over you bottom set of teeth and open and close your mouth slowly twenty times, feeling the pull along the throat. This exercise will firm up your jaw line.

- Keeping lips together, smile, pulling your smile up as high as it will go; hold for forty seconds and then release. Repeat five times. This exercise will tighten the facial muscles.

- Place your bottom set of teeth in front of the top row of teeth and smile, holding for forty seconds, then release. Repeat five times. This exercise will firm your chin.

- Place fingertips on your eyebrows. Close your eyes tightly, hold for forty seconds and release. Repeat five times. Good exercise for 'sagging' eyelids.

Repeat the above every day and you should notice a difference within a month – well, that's what the article said – and don't practise while driving the car; you may get more than you bargained for.

While we are on the subject of toning and firming, don't forget the pelvic floor exercises. These can be tightened while driving and as often as you like; only you will know why you are smiling. Chin up, girls! (Both of them.)

---

[13] Helen Evans, 'Simple ways to battle those lines', *Gulf Daily News*, 1 December 2003.

Finally, a smart blonde joke...

A blonde walks into a bank in New York City and asks for the loan officer. She says she's going to Europe on business for two weeks and needs to borrow $5,000.
The bank officer says the bank will need some kind of security for the loan, so the blonde hands over the keys to a new Rolls-Royce. The car is parked on the street in front of the bank, she has the title and everything checks out. The bank agrees to accept the car as collateral for the loan.
The bank's president and its officers all enjoy a good laugh at the blonde for using a $250,000 Rolls as collateral against a $5,000 loan. An employee of the bank then proceeds to drive the Rolls into the bank's underground garage and parks it there.
Two weeks later, the blonde returns to repay the $5,000 and the interest, which comes to $15.41.
The loan officer says, 'Miss, we are very happy to have had your business, and this transaction has worked out very nicely, but we are a little puzzled. While you were away, we checked you out and found that you are a multimillionaire. What puzzles us is, why would you bother to borrow $5,000?'
The blonde replies, 'Where else in New York City can I park my car for two weeks for only $15.41 and expect it to be there when I return?'

Bravo!

Culture Vulture

Regardless of culture and country of origin, all women the world over will experience menopause should they live to that point in their lives, and it is interesting to consider the differences in menopausal symptoms and to glean information from the research that might help any woman manage this transition in a life-affirming way.

If we had lived in ancient times, our average lifespan would have been about 28 years; we doubt we would have experienced menopause. By the twentieth century, our lifespan was around 48 years and in the twenty-first century we can live to a ripe old age of 80-plus. We are obviously doing something right, otherwise we would not have the longer lifespan. According to Thomas Perls, a geriatrician at Harvard Medical School, a woman's lifespan depends on the balance of two forces. One is the evolution drive to pass on her genes; the other is the need to stay healthy enough to rear as many children as possible. 'Menopause draws a line between the two,' he says. It protects older women from the risks of bearing children late in life and lets them live long enough to take care of their children and grandchildren. That, to us, makes sense, but the researchers in natural sciences are still puzzled by the fact that women go through menopause; that is, why nature imposed infertility on human females over an extended period in which they are not affected by senility. We think Thomas Perls answers that question.

Before we begin our cultural journey, let us sample some cultural myths. In ancient times, many traditional rituals involved the intake of menstrual blood to increase spiritual power. In ancient Greece, for example, spring festivals involved the spreading of corn and menstrual blood on the ground to increase fertility.

The word 'ritual' comes from '*rtu*', which is Sanskrit for 'menses'. Blood from the womb was believed to have the power of life. Blood sacrifices, at one time, came from the 'sacrificed' blood flow of a woman's monthly cycle. This ritual was later twisted into killing for sacrificial blood.

A woman's bleeding was once considered a powerful cosmic event connected to the lunar cycle and the tides. This connection to the moon's cycle was later misrepresented, and the connection between the wisdom of women and the tides was defamed. The word 'lunacy' is the result of this denigration.

Another word connecting women and mental instability is the word 'hysteria'. It comes from the Greek word 'hystera', meaning 'uterus'.

Both 'lunacy' and 'hysteria' are words rooted in the prevention of the female's natural reproductive cycle, and they are both terms still listed in encyclopaedias and medical dictionaries.

The word 'menopause' was first used in 1812 by a French physician named de Gardanne. At that time, it was believed that a women's mental state was directly linked to her reproductive organs. The uterus and ovaries were frequently removed as a treatment for symptoms as simple as irritability. (Phew… thank goodness we were not around then!)

Fast forward to the twentieth century: in the 1950s, we had lobotomies and female castrations as a treatment for 'midlife crazies', and by 1960 menopause was characterised as a medical disease. Which brings us to the twenty-first century, and 'menopause' is finally recognised as a natural process in a woman's life.[14]

How a woman feels during the transition to post-

---

[14] With thanks to Ms Marleen M Qunit for allowing us to use parts of her article.

menopause over a period of weeks, months or years may vary tremendously. Night sweats are a source of bother and irritability one day and absent on other days, thereby causing feelings to swing back and forth like a pendulum on a clock.

All women who are experiencing a natural menopause, as opposed to a medical or drug-induced menopause, enter peri-menopause at about the same age – 40 to 55 – all over the world, but the severity of the symptoms differ. Eastern women appear to suffer less than Western women, and the type and occurrence of symptoms women exhibit during peri-meno-pause and menopause are often related to cultural background. For instance, the hot flush is the most common symptom of Western women; however, hot flushes are so uncommon in Japan that there is no Japanese word for them. Only 24% of Eastern women suffer with hot flushes, while the figure rises to 70% of Western women; this is a huge difference. Is it only because of our cultural background?

Many Eastern women have very little knowledge about the peri-menopause symptoms, and both rural and urban women may see menopausal complaints as normal day-to-day aches and pains, even though they may have quite severe symptoms. Does this lack of awareness suggest that Eastern women are less likely to seek advice about the menopause from a medical professional than Western women?

It has yet to be determined whether peri-menopausal women from different parts of Asia suffer from the same variety of acute symptoms as Western women do, as many of the women who do go to the doctor's with symptoms such as bone pain are considered to have rheumatism and are treated for that, while depression, tension, stress, mood swings and sleeping problems are treated with tranquillisers and/or sleeping pills. Do doctors in these places have knowledge of menopause symptoms? Or do they also see it as a natural transition for a woman and think that therefore she should get on with it? Information gathered about the peri-menopause years will not be accurate if women do not recognise their symptoms as being part of their fertile decline or, due to lack of education, do not take part in surveys or talk openly of such things.

We know that exercise and the food we eat affect how our bodies function, and it is well documented that Eastern women consume more soy products than Western women. Soy contains phytoestrogens and daidzein; these are chemicals that mimic and supplement the action of the body's own hormones. Oestrogen and soy products are said both to reduce menopausal symptoms and to protect the heart.

Which brings us back to why Japanese women do not have hot flushes, and one theory is their diet, which is replete with vegetables and soy, affording them a measure of protection and prevention. In addition to this, they walk more than Western women; about forty years ago in Japan, the idea was developed that walking 10,000 steps a day would help you keep fit and healthy without the need for additional exercise.

Do not think that Japanese women have no symptoms of menopause; their symptoms are merely different. According to the Japanese Menopause Society, the most common complaints among Japanese women are fatigue, shoulder stiffness and chills. HRT is taken, but is not as popular as a more traditional and safer Kampo medicine; prescriptions for HRT account for less than 2% of the estimated 20 million menopausal Japanese women, as opposed to the 25% who take HRT in America.

Japanese women enjoy the highest average longevity in the world – almost 83.8 years – and the lowest incidences of breast cancer. But Japanese immigrants to the USA increase their risk of breast cancer and acquire incidence rates similar to the American population within two generations. This suggests that risk may be linked to environmental and behavioural factors; does this statement suggest that menopausal symptoms would also increase?

Should Western women should eat more soy product and take their exercise in the form of 10,000 steps a day in order to suffer less? We, the 'baby boomers', are the largest group experiencing menopause at this time, and we are also the first generation to be exposed to radiation, chemicals like DDT, carcinogenic chemicals, commercial chemicals found in pesticides and cleaning products, etc. Are these the reasons for why the Western women suffer more severe symptoms than the Eastern women? The food Western women eat, such as chickens, are also pumped with hormones to make them grow faster. Is this causing a problem? There are so many questions to be asked when talking about menopause and environment. Somehow, we believe, it must have an effect upon women; what do you think?

Another interesting theory is that Japan's cultural respect for older people makes the menopausal transition more comfortable; the menopausal woman is moving into a place of honour, rather than being pushed aside into a place of invisibility, as frequently occurs in Western youth-oriented cultures. Research has found that, when women hold roles that they consider important, they have fewer symptoms of menopause. Women's fears and concerns about menopause also vary by culture. Muslim Arab women fear a loss of their spouses' sexual interest when they can no longer have children. Near Eastern Jews worry about a loss of physical health; European women worry about their mental health. American women fear losing control of their emotions and becoming emotional wrecks.

In the following pages, you will read about how the menopause is experienced by women in different cultures. Some of the articles have been written by women we know or know of, and others are articles we have come across. The one thing that stands out in this is that the more affluent the woman, regardless of her culture or society, the more she will know about these changes, but that does not mean she will experience any different symptoms or cope any better.

USA by B J

While women do talk about menopause to each other and with their doctors, they primarily discuss symptoms and possible medical/alternative interventions. They do not seem to discuss the implication of menopause, e.g. changing role for the woman; implications for how a woman sees herself or how men see her. Those discussions come later, in the late 1950s, early 1960s. In a way, menopause is like death; despite talking about the physical symptoms of menopause/dying, the implications about the emotions of this change are largely swept under the rug.

I have never heard men discuss menopause. The one thing that stands out about menopause in both the US and Canada is that it is the subject of jokes. Hot flushes are 'power surges', etc. The media focuses on the humour of menopause and questions of medical treatment, and otherwise ignores it. The media focuses on the young and beautiful. Those who do not fit that description are largely ignored.

Women who have a lot of faith in the medical system seem to see menopause as something that needs to be treated by a doctor. Weird. Women who have severe and/or prolonged periods of hot flushes usually seek medical help. Hormone replacement therapy (HRT) has been associated with a number of physical diseases, and information on this is given to people by their doctors. While there are still many who choose this route, I believe there has been a decrease in its use.

However, post-menopause is also a time when women begin to find their own power. This comes from their own journey and with the support of other post-menopausal women.

Menopause is an important life passage. In many cultures, it is celebrated. North Americans are afraid of ageing and death. Exploration of the meaning and implications of menopause would be a tremendous gift to this culture. I think that the North American view of menopause is also tied into the view of women. Certainly, in the USA, women are still in a second-class position. Canada is a little further ahead in that women are accepted in powerful political positions, for example. Ultimately, the story is about how women see and value themselves, as well as society's understanding of partnership and employing the strengths of both male and female members. Changes continue to come.

Turkey by S W

Turkey is a country of diversity. Like everything else, the place of women in society stretches between two extremes. On one hand, you see the educated, highly progressed modern woman, and on the other hand there is a percentage of women who are illiterate. The social life runs parallel to the education level of women and men: on one hand, you see the modern families, both wife and husband working and having equal status in the household, and on the other hand there is the paternal family type, where the father is the head of the family and the male is dominant, even if the females of the household (wife and daughters) are working.

The modern and educated women live mainly in the big cities and are usually working. Having their financial independence and social insurance, as well as a modern outlook on life, makes it normal for them to seek help for their problems. However, not everyone does. I was reading somewhere recently that only about 10% of the female population actually do so.

Educated, working women living in the cities are more aware of what menopause is and, with medical assistance, are able to overcome it and continue their lives. However, in the rural areas, menopause is the 'end of the road'. Women tend to take on the role of the 'matriarch' in the family. As it is very common for the whole family to live together in the rural areas – grandparents, parents, children, etc. – a woman reaching the mature menopausal age expects to rule the family and can expect to be served upon by the younger ladies. Also, in the rural areas, women sometimes have to tolerate a 'concubine' brought to the house by their husbands, usually a younger girl who will be used to satisfy the physical needs of the male where the suffering menopausal might fail to do so.

All women talk to each other about peri-menopausal symptoms. It is more common for them to talk to each other than to seek help from a doctor. The educated do seek help, and to them it does not matter if they see a male or female doctor. Then there is a less educated class who will prefer female doctors. In the rural areas, it is more often the midwife whom women seek out for help. Also, the matriarchs will talk to the younger women about their experiences with menopause.

HRT is prescribed by doctors. Although I do not have statistics as to what percentage of women do use HRT in Turkey, I would imagine it is not a great percentage, bearing in mind only about 10% seek help. The use of HRT is a debatable subject in the entire world, and, in Turkey, the educated will question it, while the more conservative will not have access to it because they will not go to the doctor for menopause.

The younger generation are more aware of alternative medicine, and the use of it in menopause will increase in the coming years. As the younger generation will purchase herbs, etc., for bettering their health and beauty, it is almost inevitable that they will continue to do so in their menopausal years. People in rural areas who are reluctant to speak to doctors will take tips from each other and will use home-made remedies.

In the cities, women have access to magazines, the Internet and clinical promotions, whereas, in the rural areas, the only means of getting news are the TV or radio. Usually, programmes for women are broadcast in the afternoon, when the rural women are in the field or attending to some other work. There are civil bodies, associations that tour the rural areas and have enlightening meetings with the villagers.

This type of 'informal' educational tour needs to be more frequent and specifically cover the subject of menopause, in women-only meetings so as not to embarrass the rural women. Again, like everything else, as the educational level of women (and men) rises in Turkey, the awareness of menopause will also rise.

Kenya

A study done by Hannah Kinoti, Leah Kirumbi and Violet Kimani, the first ever done on women and menopause in Kenya, revealed interesting trends.

Elisha Anditi is a worried man. Returning from a recent visit to Kisumu, his rural home, Anditi looks confused and disorientated. For a number of weeks, his wife has been drinking huge amounts of water at alarming frequencies. She has also been sweating profusely. 'I do not know what my wife is suffering from. She just sweats and for once she did not want anything to do with me,' says Anditi. Anditi, who works in Nairobi, believes his wife, who takes care of their home in Nyanza Province, is suffering from high blood pressure. He has sent her some tablets for high blood pressure to relieve the problem.

Unlike Anditi, Peter Kamau is enraged. 'How can my wife tell me she is off sex? At night she sweats a lot, making my sheets wet, a sign that she is ready to have sex. But when I touch her, she bounces back instantly like a ball.' A resident of Central Kenya, Kamau says in frustration: 'I do not understand my wife at all. She has regular mood swings and, if she continues acting like this, I will marry another wife who can take care of my needs.'

Hilda Ngila, now fifty years old, has a different story. 'I feel dizzy at times. At other times I have hot flushes, and most of all my knees feel weak. When the flushes come and I am in a house, I immediately open the windows. I think I am suffering from malaria, which has become chronic.'

Thousands of men and women in Kenya replay these scenes everyday. However, very few relate their strange behaviour to a sexual phase known as menopause – a time when a woman stops having menstrual periods. The age of menopause in Kenya remains unknown, as is the severity of the problem and its management. Consequently, every day, most women, especially those in the rural areas, go through life without psychological or medical help.

According to Dr Caroline Odula, who has just completed her master's thesis on menopausal problems facing women in Kenya, it affects all women from as early as age forty-two and above. The worrying thing is that most doctors also do not know how to deal with the problem.

'The experience makes you feel uncomfortable, restless and embarrassed, especially when it happens in the presence of other people. In some instances, no one can help you, not even the doctors,' says Florence Joan, who is currently going through menopause. 'Menopause has changed the way I relate to men. Me and men are like water and oil and I don't want sex no matter what,' she adds.[15]

Philippines

At the start of menstruation, we are considered to be a 'woman' already and on the first day of menstruation, we are not allowed to work in the field or farm; we are just to stay in the house to do the household chores, but we are not allowed to help with heavy things, as they say it is not good for the ovaries.

---

[15] Rosemary Okello, with kind permission.

Some women are not allowed even to have their bath on their first day of menstruation because it is said cold will get into their bodies, which is not good to their health. This was my mother's generation, and some of this is not followed any more. I am now in the third generation, where there are now some modern ways. During the first generation and in second generation, women on their pre-menopausal periods take some drinks or some herbal extract medicine to avoid ovarian problems. But women before are very conservative, sensitive and protective, even these days, especially regarding women's family moral values.

Women these days seem to seek help from the doctors more than before, and herbal medication seem to be more popular these days than conventional medicine. The media is not used as much as it could be, and it would be a great help for us women if we were given information via the media.

Being an older woman in Filipina society means being loved and respected, not only within the extended family but also by people in general. It is seen as a privilege to be offered a seat on public transport; also, having heavy loads carried and being addressed politely with 'po' (please, madam). Next to this, women come into their own as the central figure within a family and, in their role as mother and grandmother, being sought as a source of advice. Getting older is seen as an unavoidable part of life and welcomed.[16]

United Kingdom

British women do seek help if needed and they do speak to each other openly about the menopause. They also don't mind if the doctor is female or male. HRT treatment is still popular, but alternative therapy is being more widely used than, say, ten years ago. Some of the differences between the

---

[16] Fe Babiano.

lower and upper classes are that the lower have less education and the upper don't really talk about it. They also think there should be more information in the doctor's clinic about menopause. Education about the menopause should also start in school, which is not widely done at the moment. [Interesting point.][17]

Holland

Menopause gets a lot of attention, especially/mainly in the magazines that target 'middle-aged women'. Women are informed of what to expect and what to do about it if they have difficulties, but it is not a subject of discussion at get-togethers, for instance; I don't know whether most middle-aged women I am close to have been through menopause already or not. I don't believe the 'value' of a woman changes in Holland if they are not fertile any more.

Early menopause is sometimes also discussed, as more women 'plan' children at an older age (late thirties).[18]

Thailand

We approached a group of five Thai ladies and asked them about menopause; they all shied away and did not like to talk about it. Then one of them told us, 'We don't speak about this; we are too shy to; not even our mothers talk to us about it. In some cases, these days, the younger generation do talk to each other about it, but in a very secret way.'

Canada

I talked to a couple of women who had already started the menopausal period of their lives, trying to get an under-

---

[17] Susan Neal.
[18] Marin Bokma.

standing of the symptoms. I also spoke to doctors, both men and women, in the hope of understanding exactly what was happening. It was hard to get an exact answer, as everyone had different symptoms and/or ideas.

I found the women who had experienced symptoms the most helpful. The male doctors were just repeating what books and lectures say, and the female doctor advised what the books say and added that, as she had not experienced menopausal symptoms, she could only repeat what she had learned through her readings.

From my talks with friends, I found my symptoms were quite mild. I did have night sweats and I asked for some help. I attended a women's health clinic and was advised to take HRT. I ran into some complications and stopped taking HRT. I discovered that I had fibroids and, after almost a year of no periods, I started having severe periods again while on HRT. Also, the controversy had started about the drug and strokes and, as I have hypertension, it was decided to stop the treatment. The doctors were starting to give me advice on alternative medicines when we moved to Bahrain. I did ask my doctor here and was told that Bahrain offered very little to menopausal women. It was almost as if you ceased to exist as a person once you longer produced, in my opinion.

HRT is still popular in Canada and it is still offered. However, I think fewer women are taking it since the uproar about its side effects or possible effects. I believe that more women are looking for alternatives to HRT or putting up with the various symptoms. I feel that it depends on the severity of the symptoms.

In Canada, I would have to say that the woman's role does not change. In some ways, it gives her more freedom. For those taking the pill, it means no more pills, no more worries. There are some symptoms with menopause that need some attention (such as vaginal dryness), but there are many products out there that help. I also think you need to keep an open dialogue with your partner, letting him/her know the problems you are experiencing.

There is a difference between classes in Canada, the same as any other country. I think the facilities are out there, but, because of the different levels of society, they are not available to all. Not all people have access to computers, so any information available on the Internet is cut off from these people. I think the middle to upper classes have more information available to them because (i) they have more education and therefore have more knowledge about themselves; (ii) they have the funds required to be 'connected'; and (iii) I think the women in these classes take more care and time for themselves. There are more speciality clinics being set up to aid all women (of all classes), but more for the lower class. Hopefully, this will put more women at ease, as they can now attend a 'women's clinic' for their problems. I don't think that there is much information available, but at least it is a start. I think a lot of women do not have many people with whom they can openly discuss their pre-menopausal concerns, and this can only improve.

I don't think there is any coverage on the topic of menopause available. There are some pamphlets available from the doctor, but these usually cover only one topic. There is not a whole lot of information over the net, either. So, on the whole, I would say that media coverage is almost non-existent. I think it would help to start putting out advice long before women reach the menopause stage. It would be helpful if you had more information at your fingertips before you really needed it. I realise that everyone has different symptoms and not everyone goes through the same thing, but I think it would be a good idea to have some facts going into the 'change'.

I would like to see some forums on the subject with both young and middle-aged women attending, with some there to relate their symptoms and experiences and some trying to figure out where they will go next. I think Canada has come quite a way, but we still need some improvements on the information road.[19]

Religious Views

Possibly because we live in an Islamic society and accept that the religious outlook is more apparent than in many Western cultures, we wanted to know how different religions view the end of a woman's fertility and her role as an elder. Below are the replies we received from different religious groups.

BUDDHISM

> In all my years of studying Buddhism, I've never heard anything about menopause. Buddhism is concerned with helping us attain liberation from suffering. Menopause is a natural function and doesn't have to do with religion as far as I'm concerned.[20]

(This is a man's answer!)

CHRISTIANITY

> Ecclesiastes 3:1 says, 'There is a time for everything, and a season for every activity under heaven.' Menopause is a season, not a disease. It's not fatal. In fact, it's a good time to take stock. In the same way that a harsh winter is always followed by spring and new life, menopause can be a precursor to a fresh beginning to the rest of your life. Take time to reflect on what you did right the first two-thirds of your life – and dare to dream about your next twenty-five or so years![21]

---

[19] Janis W.
[20] Ven Chodron.
[21] Verla Gillmor, Chicago.

ISLAM by Professor Hassan Hathout

The word menopause literally means cessation of the menstrual function, and is only a single incident along a broader complex of changes as the woman grows older, referred to as the 'climacteric', which spans perhaps several years. As normal menstrual function is the expression of cyclic hormonal changes associated with ovulation, it follows that the menopause usually heralds cessation of the reproductive function. The human female is almost unique among mammals in that her reproductive life does not continue all through her biological life, and it is not uncommon for women to have more than one third of their lives after the menopause.

Perhaps God's wisdom saw that woman's life should not be totally occupied with reproduction. Women who are post-menopausal may choose whether to fully cover themselves or not and for 'Such elderly women as are past the prospect of marriage, there is no blame on them if they lay aside their (outer) garments, provided they make not a wanton display of their beauty: but it is best for them to be modest, and God is One who sees and knows all things.' (24:60)

In communities where strong family ties still exist, it is a highly-regarded value to extend tender loving care to an old parent. The case is not so in many societies, and ageing has to be endured either in the prison of individual loneliness or in an old people's home.

Note: Any bleeding occurring during HRT treatment is considered as a nuisance to prayer activities. As a matter of fact, bleeding of this sort is different from the bleeding caused by menstruation During menstruation, prayer is not justifiable. When menstruation has ended, women take a ritual bath, *ghusl*, where the body is bathed in water and made clean. Women who menstruate should not perform *Hajj* or *umra* and they are not required to fast during Ramadan. Bleeding caused by HRT use can be justified while performing prayer. For the above rezones, it is common for women to take the contraceptive pill to avoid menstrual bleed while performing *Hajj*, *umra* and during Ramadan.[22]

JUDAISM

In general, every time period in one's life relates to another stage of potential. Just as there is tremendous beauty and possibility for a woman when she menstruates and is able to go to the mikvah, so too there is tremendous beauty when she no longer has to go to mikvah. When a woman has reached menopause, we are taught that all that is required is one final time at the mikvah to remain in the state of purity and holiness for the rest of the life. It is considered therefore a very beautiful time of life. (*Mikvah* is a beautiful ritual purifying bath.)[23]

Many traditional religions minimise the role of sexuality and limit sexual intercourse to only being permitted for procreation. With the definitive end of fertility at the time of the menopause, this gives the impression that sexuality and sexual intercourse become less important with ageing. However, physical contact should always be part of a loving relationship between a man and a woman.

A thought: humans are born virgins; we women reproduce, and then we are infertile. We have already seen that, as humans, we are very different to most mammals with regard to not being able to naturally conceive until death. We know that the lining of the vagina is thinner and, for many, the lack of sex drive means celibacy. Are we, in effect, being returned to a virginal state prior to death?

---

[22] With thanks to Sajida Adam for pointing us in the right direction.
[23] Sara Esther Crispe, Editor, TheJewishWoman.org.

What's Up, Doc?

Osteoporosis

Written by Dr Emil Hanna, Consultant Physical Medicine, Rheumatology and Rehabilitation, International Hospital, Kingdom of Bahrain

Osteoporosis is a disease of bones that makes them more fragile, so eventually they can be broken very easily. The bones that are most likely to be broken in patients with osteoporosis are the hip, the bones above the wrist joint and the vertebrae. When vertebra are affected, people with osteoporosis lose height and their back becomes severely curved and hunched.

Unfortunately, this disease develops painlessly, so people with this disease do not know about it until they break a bone; this is why it is called the 'silent thief'.

Women are at a higher risk of developing osteoporosis because they have lower bone mass and hence weaker bones than men of the same age. Postmenopausal women are more likely to develop osteoporosis due to loss of oestrogen, which keeps the strength of their bones.

Some diseases increase the risk of developing osteoporosis, such as an overactive thyroid gland and anorexia nervosa. Patients who receive cortisone medications are at a higher risk as well.

Here are some ways to keep our bones in the best of health and help you live longer:

1. *See your doctors if you are at risk of osteoporosis.*
    - If your menopause occurred before the age of 45 or you have had a hysterectomy or an operation to remove your ovaries.
    - If osteoporosis runs in your family.
    - If you are underweight or slender-built.
    - If you have taken steroid medicines for a long period of time.
    - If you have ever broken a bone as a result of a minor fall or injury.

2. *Test your bone density.*
    - The most reliable and the most popular test is bone densitometry (DEXA). It is very safe because it uses a very low amount of X-rays. 'DEXA test is recommended to be done yearly.'

3. *Exercise regularly.* Take weight-bearing exercise such as brisk walking, running, aerobics and tennis. Try to exercise for twenty minutes at least three times a week. If you have been told that you have osteoporosis, avoid exercise that:
    - Involves strong sudden movements, such as squash or badminton;
    - Puts excessive strain on a part of your body (e.g. sit-ups);
    - May cause you to fall suddenly.

4. *Quit now.* If you are a smoker, give up. Smoking has a toxic effect on your bones; it may also increase the risk of hip fracture later in life. So, in addition to your heart, lungs and circulation, your bones are another part of your body that will benefit if you stop smoking.

5. *Avoid alcohol intake.* Alcohol can reduce calcium absorption and can affect bone growth.

6. *Get enough calcium.* If there is little calcium in your diet, you may be depriving your bones of the essential mineral that they require to stay strong. The best sources are milk and dairy products, such as yoghurt and cheese. You can also get it from leafy vegetables.

7. *Get enough vitamin D.* You can get vitamin D from sunlight (just five to ten minutes a day). Vitamin D is needed to absorb calcium and turn it into bone. Certain foods, including salmon, sardines, egg yolk, cod liver oil and dairy products, are good sources of vitamin D. If you are at risk of osteoporosis or you are elderly, you can benefit from vitamin D supplements.

8. *Forget the fizz.* Sweet fizzy drinks contain the preservative phosphoric acid, which, if consumed in excess, can disrupt the balance of calcium in the body.

9. *Reduce the likelihood of having a fall.*

   • Get your eyes tested; good vision means you are less likely to trip up over unseen obstacles.

   • Remove obstacles at home that might trip you up (such as loose carpets and small furniture).

   • Use some sort of support (stick or walking frame) to aid your balance as you walk if you have difficulties with walking or balance.

10. *Don't despair – medical treatment is available.*

    • Hormone replacement therapy (HRT) replaces oestrogen that the body stops producing at menopause.

    • Alendronate (Foamex) is a non-hormonal medicine used once weekly that prevents bone loss.

    • Calcium hormone.

    • Calcium and vitamin D supplements, if needed.

Remember, if your bones are healthy, there are steps you can take to keep them that way.

Nutritional Advice for Menopause

*Written by Dr Neriman Rashad Ali Lotfi, MBBS, DIP, Msc
General Practitioner and Clinical Nutritionist*

During my years in practice many women have come to see me for pre- and post-menopausal problems. But it concerns me that the women of today still feel embarrassment, discomfort, and even denial when talking about menopause. So, when I was approached by Kate and Maggie to write an article, I was more than happy to do so.

Staying healthy during and after menopause may mean making some changes in the way you live, such as:

- Eating a healthy, balanced diet, which is low in fat, high in fibre, and contains fresh fruits, vegetables and whole-grain foods.

- Limiting saturated fats, refined sugars and processed foods.

- Making sure you are getting your vitamins and minerals; aim for 1,500 milligrams of calcium and 400 to 800 international units of vitamin D a day. Ask your doctor about supplements to help you meet these requirements, if necessary.

- Learn what your healthy weight is, and try to maintain that weight.

- Do your regular annual check-up to maintain healthy blood pressure and blood cholesterol levels.

- Exercise regularly, do some cardiovascular exercises, such as walking, jogging, cycling or dancing, at least three days each week for a healthy heart, and combine it with some weight-bearing exercises, as these help to increase bone density and reduce the chance of getting osteoporosis. Try to be physically active in other ways as well, such as taking the stairs instead of a lift or parking your car further away from your destination; the extra walk will also help your general health.

Findings from research suggest that regular exercise programmes can help to alleviate some of the physical symptoms associated with the menopause and improve a woman's health and quality of life. Exercise will also help you if you have sleeping problems, and it is one of the best methods of fighting post-menopausal depression. Personally, I like to see exercise programmes offered by primary healthcare professionals for menopausal women.

Many women use natural product supplements, but be sure to consult your doctor before taking any herbal treatments or dietary supplements for signs and symptoms of menopause. Herbal products can interfere or interact with other medications you may be taking.

It is very important that you drink a sufficient amount of water per day to make up for fluids lost. The benefits of drinking water are widely recognised. Drinking pure, fresh water is essential to our health and well-being; as we grow older, our need for fresh water increases. Our skin and mucus membranes become thinner and lose more water; also, our kidneys function less efficiently as we age. Did you know that the average amount of water loss per day is two cups through breathing, two cups through invisible perspiration, and six cups through urination and bowel movements? That is a total of ten cups lost per day without taking into account perspiration from exercise or hard work, excessively dry air, alcohol and caffeine consumption. You may not feel thirsty, but you should get into the habit of drinking water, nevertheless.

Last but not least is smoking: it's never too late to quit smoking. We all know that smoking increases your risk of heart disease, stroke, cancer and a range of other health problems. It may also increase hot flushes and bring on earlier menopause. And you have also now reached the age where all of these illnesses are at high risk, so why jeopardise your life by smoking?

I would also like to address stress, which is also very common during this stage in your life; the important thing is to learn how to control the stress and relax.

- Change your thinking: reframe your thoughts; try to think more positively and be optimistic.

- Change your behaviour: be assertive, get organised, have fun, diversify and let yourself be distracted; day-dreaming can be a therapeutic release.

- Change your lifestyle: try meditation, deep breathing, yoga, massage, nature walks, music, and get enough sleep every day, since exhaustion reduces your ability to face or overcome stress.

Finally, many women find that, with the cessation of their monthly cycle, a new phase of life begins; enjoy the woman you have now become.

Questions and Answers

When we initially decided to write a book about menopause, we were not too sure of the direction it would take. We knew what we wanted to cover and decided that, by sending out a questionnaire, we could get insight on how women feel about being 40-plus, the 'change' of their lives and the future.

Luckily, the replies did answer some questions for us, as well as giving us a few surprises. Now that we ourselves know more about this time in our lives, we would probably have asked a few different questions.

Below is a copy of the questionnaire that we sent out. A total of 68 women took the time to read, digest and reply, and for your time and cooperation, ladies, we are grateful.

Questionnaire

Name (optional)	
Age	
Nationality	
Country of Residence	
If this is not your country of birth, do you think your life is better in your country of residence than it would be in your native country?	

Marital Status	Married □	Life Partner □	Single □	Divorced □	Widow □
If divorced, how many marriages?					
Work experience	Employer □	Employee □		Home-maker □	Other □
Family Income	Low □		Medium □		High □
Children, how many?					
Diet	Vegan □	Vegetarian □	Red Meat and Fish □		White Meat and Fish □
How often do you eat fruit?	Daily □	Weekly □	Now and Then □		Never □
Exercise?	None at All □		Regular □		Sporadic □
Please specify					
Do you take any supplements?	Vitamins □		Minerals □		HRT □
Please specify					
What did you feel about approaching 40?					
Do you feel 40+ is middle-aged?	Yes □			No □	
Do you see a man as being middle-aged at 40+?	Yes □			No □	
Any changes, e.g. physical, emotional, mental, metabolism, sex drive after turning 40?					
Do you speak openly about the menopause ?	Friends □		Doctors □		None □

If not, please specify		
Do you feel the media has influenced how you see yourself? Positively or negatively?		
Are you more likely to buy age-defying products that you see advertised?	Yes □	No □
Have you had or would you consider having Botox injections or cosmetic surgery?		
What is the up-side to being 40-plus? And the downside?		
What are your fears?		
How do you see the future?		

Questionnaire Responses

We made the decision not to put the answers in a 'table' format because, as you will see, some of the questions could be answered with a 'yes' or 'no', while other questions have comments added; some are just one word, others a sentence, and we think it is inspiring to read the answers as they were given.

If this is not your country of birth, do you think your life is better in your country of residence than it would be in your native country?

- 98% of the women resided in their native country. The remaining 2% felt life was better as an expat.

Exercise?

- None at all, 7%,

- Regular, 63%,

- Sporadic, 29%,

- No answer, 1%.

Do you take any supplements?

- 20% of the women were on HRT.

- Supplements regularly taken included cod liver oil, evening primrose, echinacea, multivitamins, spirulina, B complex, vitamin A, C, D, E, multi-minerals, flax-seed, Centrum, salmon oil, coenzyme Q10, calcium, anti-oxidant, garlic, cultrate, silica, iron, Omega 3, magnesium, folic acid, glucosamine, zinc, vegEPA.

What did you feel about approaching 40?

Positive

- Life begins.
- Happy in my 40s.
- Totally relaxed.
- No bother at all.
- Achieved a lot.
- Wonderful.
- Excitement.
- Good.
- Small things do not mean much any more.
- Pizza and champagne at Twin Palms!
- No worries, I was looking forward to giving birth to my third child.
- No problems – it was just about the happiest time in my life, so 40 just slipped by!
- Didn't trouble me, I still had plenty of energy and didn't feel as if I were getting older.
- Looking forward, because I feel better and better every year.

Negative

- Awful.
- Did not like it.

Grey Area

- Nothing.
- Normal, no fears.

- Happened very quickly.

- Scary at first, then feeling calmer.

- Not an issue, wonder what the fuss is all about.

- Lots of changes, I did not know what to expect.

- I must admit that it really did not bother me – I think approaching 60 is much more daunting.

- Old age is much closer and you really do look at how you are going to spend the remaining part of your life and try to fit in all the things you really want to do before the ability to do things is taken away from you.

- OK, but did not like getting older.

- Who has the time to think when you have three children?

- Did not have a problem with 40, but 49 was a real trip. By 50 I had already gotten over it from stressing the whole 49th year.

- Did not think much about it until arrived and then I wanted to hide the age or lie about it.

- Did not feel much different apart from hot flushes, aches and pains and greying!

Any changes, e.g. physical, emotional, mental, metabolism, sex drive after turning 40?

Physical

Positive

- Nothing.

- Relaxed with my body.

- Kids keep me young.

- Good.

- I don't remember too many outstanding issues at turning 40; I guess I still had too much on my plate with job, children, house, etc.

- I did not have many side-effects from the change of life, and by 55 I was basically done.

- I hear stories of women having a terrible time, but I guess I was one of the lucky ones.

Negative

- Weight gain.

- Gravity took over.

- All downhill.

- Memory lapses.

- Just prefer to sleep.

- Physically tired.

- Possibly more tired, but I don't want to get older now.

- How many pages do you want? I put on weight much more easily and it is hard to get it off.

- Brain wants to do things, but body does not have as much energy as before. It is all downhill from 35. Aches and pains seems to start at 45 or so.

- More tired and nod off on the sofa in the evening.

Grey Area

- Wearing glasses. Gradual changes.

- Start looking my age.

- No; some of those things came when I was into my 50s.

- I wasn't aware of any particular changes until after I was 57. Since then it has been mainly a decline in energy levels.

- I took HRT for about 4 years but stopped because I was horrified how it was made. Also by that time, research did seem to say that maybe it was not so great after all. Looking back, it probably helped hot flushes as I cannot remember having any until much later, and boy did I suffer – drenched – and that still happens occasionally.

- There were no marked changes in my life because of it.

Emotional

- Grateful. Fitting into my own skin.

- Yes. I felt more need to be pampered.

- Depressed at turning 40, started on antidepressants.

- I originally started HRT, as I was terribly up and down in moods and temper; certainly helped. When I stopped the HRT, I began using progesterone cream – a bit of a faff both to get and to use. I am not convinced it helped. After a few years I stopped everything and felt no worse.

Mental

- More assertive.

- Confident in own abilities.

- Eager to learn from others.

- Take action.

Metabolism

- Same.

- Not working.

- Slower metabolism, harder to lose weight.

Sex Drive

- Much better.

- Got a new man in my life.

- Lost, unless George Clooney knocks on my door.

- Improved.
- Waves of rampant desire and waves of preferring a good book.
- Higher than ever.
- Bit of a problem with vaginal dryness.
- Sex drive not as much either. Improved at the age 49–50.
- Sex got better when was on HRT. Skin better. Not so much vaginal soreness with sex and produced more lubricant.
- No real change/great relief at not having to worry about pregnancies, so probably made it better! Pity about not being able to stay awake!

Do you speak openly about the menopause?

- 74% spoke to both friends and doctors.
- 5%, doctors only.
- 7%, friends only.
- 0%, no one.
- 14%, did not answer.

Comments

- Friend discussions not a big issue for me personally yet, but have been an area of concern and discussions for other friends and my mother.
- I am grateful to be alive.
- Do not feel it's taboo subject, but I think we can get caught up in ourselves too much.
- We only have a God-given day at a time and some of the most wonderful people I know are too busy thinking of others to tune in too much – but when it happens I think it effects those around us as much as ourselves.

- This is an area I hope to accept when it appears – on the outside, I believe, I want to look no older, and on the inside I hope to feel pretty much as I do now.

- I was very lucky and had few problems.

- Have not needed to discuss menopause with doctors at this point. I may be in 'pre' but not sure.

- No real symptoms at this time (I'm 50) – but Mom didn't start menopause till she was 52.

Do you feel the media has influenced how you see yourself? Positively or negatively?

Comments

- Choose not to watch TV & listen to radio.

- Isn't 40 the new 30?

- Positive.

- Don't read that literature.

- That's their job.

- Combination of both.

- I like myself.

- I don't know, I think the media today present women as still young at 40.

- Media have a more negative view of 40-plus than I have.

- Everybody should look thin and skinny.

- Media still tries to make us believe that slim is beautiful. I am not slim, I am positive.

- Stereotyping is very wrong for the young. It is the beauty within that attracts me to people, and I want to be around people who grow and develop through life's experience.

- I don't buy magazines, because I believe I would become discontent with overexposure to advertising and chasing youth culture.

- No. I think that a lot of media hype is mainly some form of advertisement and pay little attention to it.

- I think media has improved in the last few years, as the more mature women seem to have a place – of course, they have discovered that we have the money to spend. But we are still youth-obsessed, I think.

- The media is doing a better job at making you believe it is OK to get older.

- It is helping teach people to take better care of themselves.

- I think they realise that in America, at least, very soon there will be more 'older' people than younger people, due to the baby boomers coming of age.

- I don't take much notice of media issues, I'm my own person – please myself.

- I get influenced but try to stay away.

- It forces me to take better care of my body so I get better looks.

- Not too bothered about what media has to say about being over 40.

Are you more likely to buy age-defying products that you see advertised?

- Yes, 68%

- No, 14%,

- No answer, 6%

Comments

- Don't buy them.

- Some.

- I worked in advertising and know what baloney it is.
- Yes, absolutely – for health reasons and skin mostly.
- My body is going to do what it is going to do.
- Somehow you find the cash when you want to put off the ageing process.

Have you had or would you consider having Botox injections or cosmetic surgery?

- Yes, 20%
- No, 80%

Comments

- Would never do plastic surgery or expensive procedures.
- Still sceptical, had friends who have succumbed.
- Had money = tummy tuck & lower eye bags.
- Botox = migraine control.
- Correct acne-damage rather than wrinkles.
- Not at the moment.
- Scared of doing it.
- Only if I had an accident and looked like a monster.
- What you see is what you get.
- I have grown children, so who am I kidding?
- Again, I am quite comfortable with who I am and what I look like.
- No – too dangerous.
- Only thing would be boob lift after losing weight (maybe) and maybe a tummy tuck.
- Certainly not! I would consider it an utter waste of money. I'd rather have a new ring.

- No to Botox – would not mind having eyes and chin done if money was no object.
- I have not had but maybe some day; not Botox, but surgery.
- Absolutely not! Grow old gracefully is my motto.

What is the upside to being 40-plus. And the downside?

Upside

- Life journey. Life is more stable. More self-assured. More decisiveness and self-assurance.
- Satisfied with my life, done a lot. Feeling comfortable with myself. Finally my time had come.
- Peace with myself. No fear of pregnancy. Having good friends. You are smarter and more experienced.
- Have learned hard lessons. More confident in who I am – comfortable being me.
- Acceptance of a day at a time. Finished most of my responsibilities. Lucky staying healthy at this age.
- That I am grateful to be here with a love of life. Being wiser and more tolerant.
- Fewer money worries and children worries. Learning to like yourself and accepting who you are.
- Freedom from periods and all that mess. Felt more at one with myself. Calmer, don't put as high demands on myself any more.
- Feel more experienced, content and aware of self; looking forward to doing more.
- I have paid my dues to society in terms of work and volunteering.
- Age 40 marked the moment when I began to pursue my own interests.

- This was an entry into my self-empowerment, which was and continues to be magnificent.

- Fewer demands from family members, so more free time.

- Understanding who you are and not putting up with the crap one was once forced to do on the way up the proverbial ladder of life.

- More convinced; dare to be yourself; want to try doing more things and achieve; accept things easily.

- I had reached the maturity I wanted, but people around regarded 40-plus as becoming old.

- That my children have grown and left the nest and now it is my husband and I to do the things that we want.

- One feels more confident, less pressure from children.

- Look forward to retirement, but always worry whether there will be enough money.

- Pleasure from our daughters, maturity and acceptance of 'where I'm at'.

- Not worrying too much about what other people think about you; far more confident and happy in my skin.

- Self-confidence; I know what I want; other listens more; don't care that much what others say.

- Your family is growing up and you can get on with your life.

- Don't take things so seriously; if you have been taking care of husband, children, job, housework, then you can manage everything else.

- Have done what I had to do, now new opportunity doors open.

- Being part of the fixture and fittings at work and feeling comfortable with that.

Downside

- More tired. Tired feet. Money. More crow feet! Memory problems. Less time to live. Losing confidence.

- It's near 50 and 60. All downhill from here. Less fit. Getting older and stiff. Reduced energy levels.

- The body will soon say stop. Aches and pains increase. I don't like mirrors any more. Hate age spots and purple spots.

- Night sweats and hot flushes. Not being able to fulfil all ambitions. Not recovering as quickly from colds and flu.

- Not feeling quite so useful any more. Not being successful with job applications.

- Unstable feet – falling down, breaking bones easier. Forgetfulness and dementia and kids talking down to you.

- Have to slow down with my daily work. I feel young inside but look old outside. Loss of skin tone, muscle tone.

- Don't like looking older and minor ageing complaints. I don't fit the things I wore when I was 20.

- I don't have time and money to do all I like. Realising that your body is going to disappoint you.

- Wished that I had been more aware and started my path earlier.

- I can see my mother getting older and know it won't be long until I am there.

- If not married or with a partner you are classed as 'too old' and it's hard to find a male to be interested in you when there is plenty of young blood around.

- Society sees you as old, body slows down and you can't do all that your mind thinks it can do.

- Clothes in magazines only for slim young people; magazines do not really cater for our age.

- We now have parents to look after, so we are not as free as we would like.

- I find it humorous and often say, 'Oh no, I am turning into my mother.' And I *am*!

- Not having quite the same energy and power and everything finding its way south!

- Of course things are progressing as far as age goes.

- Grey hair, lines and wrinkles, sagging boobs and bums that will hit the floor, tummies that you can't see your feet below, not being quite so energetic.

What are your fears?

- Loneliness. Family health. Looking old. Losing loved ones. Getting less mobile. Losing mental faculties.

- None. Physical disability. Getting priorities out of order. Being alone. Being too old to drive safely.

- Long-term ill health, not being mobile, getting fat.

- Snakes and being alone in a home.

- I am not afraid any more.

- Don't think I really have any.

- No fears as long as I am with my family.

- Losing my parents, as I know I will.

- My mother-in-law outliving me, the old witch.

- Alzheimer's (crosswords, Sudoku hopefully will help keep it away).

- Having poor health just when I want to go forward.

- Wrinkles, flab, any kind of incapacitation.

- To be really sick and to lose one of my children or my husband.

- That anyone in my family dies before me, mostly my children.

- Running out of time and not seeing my children grow up.

- Losing loving relationship that I share with my husband.

- Worry about old age and being a burden when very old.

- Having enough money for a long and healthy retirement.

- Running out of time before I complete the several lifetimes of learning and experience I have planned for this life.

- Don't really have any – would wish for continued happiness and contentment and would hope to maintain reasonable health until I fall off my perch!

- Being looked after by the kids in my old age.

- World – enough food for the starving.

- People getting along together in harmony.

How do you see the future?

- Full of possibility. Promising. With curiosity. Very positive.

- Good, bright and exciting. Look forward to it.

- Optimistically. It's only getting better. Keep fit, stay happy.

- Time to travel, etc. As a room full of open doors.

- God-given, a day at a time.

- Time for hobbies and interests.

- Future is good if health is good.

- Positive as long as I am healthy.

- I am a positive person, so with optimism.

- An active 60- to 70-year-old biking in Bali!

- I like the expression 'Don't worry, be happy'.

- Future will be what I make it to be.

- Live to the full, be positive, learn.

- Not having to be so dynamic.

- Not being stressed or rushing around as much.

- In my control and therefore bright.

- Contentment, togetherness time with husband, home, holidays (a lot of them).

- Think positive, easy life; don't worry and be happy.

- I am positive about the future – life is good.

- Try to remain optimistic but do have concerns as I believe most thinking people do, e.g. global warming, selfish attitudes of society, the future for my kids.

- Fortunately, I fell in love at 45 and found that life does not actually end once you are in your 40s.

- I feel I need a goal to work towards to give meaning to my later years.

- We started out as two and now we are back to being two; we are best friends.

- At the moment, I look forward to continuing a fulfilling and busy life. As for the world, I hope that all difficulties will be dealt with and that there will be peace for all.

As you can see from the above, women generally are positive and confident with their age and within themselves. Regardless of age, nationality, culture, wealth or diet, women experience a natural menopause at around the same ages and with much the same symptoms, although varying symptoms are experienced by most.

Once through the menopause years, life appears to hold much promise and it is rewarding to see women take life in their stride and, as most of us do, get on with it.

At the beginning of the book, we mentioned that menopause is a fairly 'new' phenomenon, as women are now living longer than previous generations. Of all of the medical problems associated with being older, it is only the menopause that can be said to affect all women, the world over, and this may be the reason we are still trying to figure out the manic hormone rampage that can make our life a misery.

In the Western, progressive societies, more women and men are experiencing fertility problems, and this is put down to environment, sexual lifestyle and nutrition as well as women and/or couples leaving the role of becoming parents to the later years – 30-plus onwards. So, if a woman's eggs and a man's sperm are no longer viable, will these women experience menopause on the same scale as today's woman and at a similar age? Another thing to consider is this: if today's children are reaching sexual maturity earlier than their predecessors, will they also decline, hormonally, at an earlier age, age prematurely and expire younger? This would be nature's way of slowing down overpopulation. We all know that the resources of this planet are finite and, even with all of the technological advances made, Mother Nature still holds the winning hand.

We doubt we will be around to witness these events, if they occur, but we will be remembered – if not by a gravestone, then by our adaptation of ageing. We have reached the end of the fertile line, but, instead of bowing gracefully to old age and death, we are taking these extra years to make a statement, even if it is only to ourselves.

Women over 40 *rock*!

Glossary

Alzheimer's	The most common cause of dementia, afflicting those in middle or old age, and a degenerative disease of the cerebral cortex for which there is no cure. Symptoms include paralysis and progressive loss of memory and speech. The cause is not understood but is the subject of ongoing research.
benign	A term used most frequently to refer to tumours, meaning 'not harmful'.
cancer	A commonly used term for any form of malignant tumour. It is characterised by an uncontrolled and abnormal growth of cancer cells, which attack nearby tissues and destroy them.
chemotherapy	A treatment of a disease by the administration of chemical substances or drugs. It includes the treatment of infectious diseases with antibiotics, and other types of drugs; also, the treatment and control of various tropical diseases and, especially in recent years, many different forms of cancer with anti-metabolite drugs.
dementia	A mental disorder typified by confusion, disorientation, memory loss, personality changes and a lessening of intellectual capacity.
endocrine system	Various endocrine glands that secrete hormones in the space outside the body cells to be passed into the blood capillaries and carried around the body by the bloodstream.

heart block

A condition in which there is a failure in the transmission of electrical impulses from the natural pacemaker (the sinoatrial node) through the heart, which can lead to a slowing of the pumping action.

heart attack

(Also: *coronary thrombosis.*) A sudden blockage of one of the coronary arteries by a blood clot or thrombus, interrupting the blood supply to the heart.

hormone therapy

(*HRT*) Some women may choose to take the hormones oestrogen and progesterone after menopause to relieve hot flushes and vaginal dryness and to protect against osteoporosis. Taking oestrogen alone increases a woman's risk of uterine cancer. Taking progesterone with oestrogen decreases the risk of uterus cancer, but it can cause bleeding in menopausal women.

hypertension

High blood pressure; refers to a condition in which the blood pumps around the body at too high a pressure.

hypotension

The medical term for low blood pressure.

hysterectomy

A surgical removal of the uterus. It is commonly carried out if fibroids are present, if the uterus is cancerous or if there is excessive bleeding. A hysterectomy may be total (removing the body and cervix of the uterus) or partial (also called supra-cervical). In many cases, surgical removal of the ovaries (oophorectomy) is performed simultaneously. The surgery is then called 'total abdominal hysterectomy with salpingo-oophorectomy'.

hysteria

A type of neurosis that is difficult to define and in which a range of symptoms may occur. These includes paralysis, seizures and spasming of limbs, swelling of joints, mental disorder and amnesia.

mammography	A special X-ray technique used to determine the structure of the breast. It is useful in the early detection of tumours and in distinguishing between benign and malignant tumours.

malignant	A term used in several ways: to describe a tumour that proliferates rapidly, destroys surrounding healthy tissues and can spread via the lymphatic system and bloodstream to other parts of the body, or to describe a form of a disease that is more serious than the usual one and is life-threatening, such as malignant hypertension.

Pap smear	A simple test involving scraping off some cells from the cervix and examining them microscopically. The test is recommended to be carried out once a year to every three years (ask for your doctor's advice) to detect early indications of cancer, and is a form of preventive medicine.

premature ovarian failure (POF)

POF is defined as menopause that occurs before the age of 40 and is not induced by a physician; in other words, it is identical to natural menopause but it occurs before the age of 40.

radiotherapy	A therapeutic use of penetrating radiation, including X-rays, beta rays and gamma rays. These may be derived from X-ray machines or radiation isotopes and are especially employed in the treatment of cancer. The main disadvantage of radiotherapy is that there may be damage to normal, healthy surrounding tissues.

thyroid	A gland situated at the base and front of the neck. It produces two hormones: thyroxine and triiodothyronine, which are essential for the regulation of metabolism and growth.

ultrasound   High-frequency sound waves, beyond the range of the human ear. Used to examine the body organs, ducts, etc., or assess the progress of a developing foetus.

Useful Web Sites

www.agepositive.gov.uk

www.agepositive.gov.uk

www.andropause.com

www.avert.org

www.careaware.co.uk

www.citizensadvice.org.uk

www.direct.gov.uk/Over50s

www.elderabuse.org.uk.

www.gynob.com/menopause

www.helptheaged.org.uk

www.heyday.org.uk

www.menstuff.org

www.saga.co.uk

www.strongwomen.com

www.wikipedia.org

Select Bibliography

AVERT, www.avert.co.uk

Chambers Dictionary, 10th edition, Chambers Harrap Publishers Ltd, 2006

Consumer Health Digest, *www.consumerhealthdigest.com*

Dove Campaign for Real Beauty, *www.campaignforrealbeauty.co.uk*

Dr Gerard DiLeo, *www.gynob.com*

Encarta Online Encyclopaedia, Dictionary, Atlas and Homework, *www.encarta.msn.com*

Helen Evans, 'Simple ways to battle those lines', *Gulf Daily News*, 1 December 2003

Woods, Judith, 'Mid-life crisis? Bring it on!', *Healthy*, Issue 42, March 2006

www.islamnet.com

9 781847 481160